Food Combining and Digestion

Food Combining and Digestion

101 Ways to Improve Digestion

by Steve Meyerowitz

Illustrations by Rick Meyerowitz

Sproutman Publications • www.Sproutman.com

Library of Congress Cataloging-in-Publication Data
Meyerowitz, Steve.
Food combining & digestion : easy to follow techniques to increase
stomach power and maximize digestion / by Steve Meyerowitz ;
illustrations by Rick Meyerowitz.
p. cm.
ISBN 1-878736-77-9
1. Food combining. I. Title: Food combining and digestion. II. Title.

RA784 .M483 2002   ₹
613.2–dc21
                        2002011246

Cover Illustration and illustrations on p.14, 20 & 36 by Rick Meyerowitz.
Illustrations on p. 34 & 101 by Michael J. Parman.
Cover design by George Foster

Disclaimer: The information in this book is for educational purposes
only. It is not medical advice, nor is it intended to replace the advice of
your physician. Consult a licensed health professional for diagnosis and
treatment of illness, for advice regarding medications, and before
making changes to your diet or exercise program.

Distributed by
Book Publishing Company
PO Box 99, Summertown, TN 38483
888-260-8458. 931-964-3571. Fax 931-964-3518
www.bookpubco.com e-mail: info@bookpubco.com

Table of Contents

Introduction

True happiness is impossible without true health and true health is impossible without a rigid control of the palate.
—Mahatma Gandhi

The Art of Food Combining

Food combining is the process of orchestrating our meals in such a way as to keep our stomachs sound and happy. No one likes a grumbling stomach and bad diet choices can absolutely ruin a good day. Gas, indigestion, distention, sour stomach, and acid reflux are all too common in modern society. Drugs to quell these complaints are among the best sellers in pharmacies.

Is It Art or Science?

Most of us think of food combining as a science governed by laws of chemistry. Protein digestion requires an acid medium, starch digestion requires alkaline enzymes, sugars like lactose require specific enzymes like lactase, and so forth. If good digestion was simply a matter of chemical combinations, we could satisfy the unanswered questions with a combining chart. Indeed, many people walk around with food combining charts in their pockets and whip them out in advance of every gulp. Although we respect the science behind food combining and abide by the chemistry involved, there are other, non-scientific, factors that play a more significant role in our effort to achieve optimum digestion.

When it comes to good digestion, everything matters. Lifestyle, emotions, attitude, timing, habits and environment all contribute to the "art" of food combining. The whole scenario of our daily lives figures into the efficiency of our stomachs. Digestion is not just getting food in and out. It is the absorption and assimilation of nutrients for the construction and repair of cells and the nourishment of the "whole" body. In one respect, this books plays the very pedestrian role of simply teaching proper eating habits. This involves not only what, where, how, when and why we eat, but also our consciousness during the process of nourishing ourselves.

Food encompasses our whole world, everything we do, everywhere we go, no matter what country or culture. Our social interactions revolve around questions of: Did you eat? What do you want to eat? Where shall we eat? When do you wish to eat? If we stop eating, the world becomes vastly different. Sadly, many people would experience how empty their lives are. Others may not know what to do with all the extra free time. Try fasting sometime and watch how the world changes.

Our bodies are endowed with miraculous equipment that can digest the worst chemical combinations as long as we do not overdo it. To achieve optimum digestion and good health, we need only to learn our limits and become more conscious of what we eat while we are eating it. Unfortunately, most of us spend so much time working that we forget our bodies and lose touch with what we put in them. Indigestion is a red flag. It tells us to slow down and watch what we are eating. We need to treat our stomachs like we would treat a baby. Be sensitive. Savor every bite–even every gulp of water! Don't worry about counting enzymes or vitamins. Our body chemistry is far too complex for our conscious minds to regulate. But we can make a difference by cultivating good eating habits and shunning bad ones. For starters, we need to eat less and our meals need to be less complex. Animals eat one food at a time. Let your goal be to simplify your meals. Eat consciously, judiciously and apply common sense. As Swami Digestananda says at the end of this book, most of all enjoy your food and be happy, then you will digest every bite.

Sproutman®

Steve Meyerowitz

The Laws of Food Combining

*The act of breaking down and digesting foods frees
the forces inherent in them, forces related to the
various complexes of organs. Material nutrients are
thus transformed into forces that nourish the
nervous system and the brain...Food is a support
that can be made use of only to the degree that the
individual spirit actively transforms it.*
—Rudolf Hauschka

You Are What You Eat

Laws? No. The human body does not operate like a govern-
ment system with political laws. But, it is a system governed by physical laws. Like any system, when these laws or limitations are
exceeded, problems occur. Most of the time, the penalties are not
immediately evident. Just like when the federal budget is out of balance, we persevere, however blindly, thanks to deficit spending.
The effects of violating this economic law will be borne largely by
the next generation. The economy may suffer with depression, in-
flation, higher taxes, or unemployment. Someone will pay.

In the same way, you may violate the "laws" of your physical
body and not "pay" until later in life—with symptoms like irritable
bowel, hypoglycemia, fibromyalgia, ulcers, arthritis, eczema, colon
cancer, etc. Some of us pay right away in the form of stomach ache,
headache, flatulence, diarrhea, or indigestion. But most of us walk
around with minor problems like these for years and pay no attention to it. Since we don't know what to do about it, we decide it is an
annoyance and ignore it. Some of us seek help, but if the doctors
can't find anything, it continues to get ignored. Conventional medical doctors are good at finding acute problems, but have difficulty
treating some of the above mentioned chronic complaints. Often,
the answer can be found in watching what we eat and how we eat it.

Many problems are related to food in some way. It's true: "we are what we eat." Even the medical profession is now beginning to recognize it. The National Cancer Institute is suggesting we all eat high fiber foods and increase our consumption of fresh fruits and vegetables. They recommend five fruit or vegetable servings every day. Whether you are 50 and have recently discovered an ulcer, or 5 and get a rash after eating citrus, there are certain digestive rules we must live by if we desire optimal health.

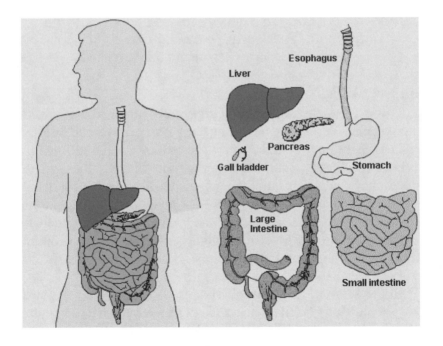

Digestion is not just getting food in and out. It is the absorption and assimilation of nutrients for the construction and repair of cells and the nourishment of the whole body.

QUANTITY
The First Law of Digestion

In general, mankind since the improvement of
cookery, eats twice as much as nature requires.

—Benjamin Franklin

Everybody has their limit. Our stomachs are merely physical systems. Like different brands of machines, they vary in size, amount of digestive juices available, strength and content of those juices and ability to replenish themselves. So, if you want to wash a big rug, you bring it to the commercial laundry because it would overtax your home washer and dryer. Machines have limitations and we would do well to think of our digestive systems as also having limitations.

People do not pay enough attention to their stomachs. Advertising fools us into believing we can consume anything. We yearn for a "whopper" of a meal. The TV jingles sing about "a double cheeseburger with pickles, onions, tomatoes, cabbage, fries, Worcestershire sauce on a sesame seed bun." That's almost too much to say—much less eat! And don't forget the large soda, malted or thick shake. Our appetites are far ahead of our stomachs. The old adage "the eyes are bigger than the stomach" is embarrassingly true. We can go a long way toward better Digestion–and better health–by remembering that we have stomachs down there that can only handle so much. Man can survive on one third of his daily food intake. The other two thirds goes to the benefit of the health insurance and medical care industries.

We are the cause of our indigestion. What if your town just had a big parade, one so large that it took a week to clean up. The townspeople would be upset because normal business and transportation would be disrupted for so long. Indeed, it may have been fun, but it was beyond the city's capacity. In the same way, you might yell at your teenager because they made a mess in their room that was impossible to clean up without help. Or you might be spending more with your credit card than you can afford to pay at the end of the month. Admittedly, we live in a deficit thinking society. But you cannot blame society for your indigestion.

We bite off more than we can chew. If we want optimum digestion and superior health, we must practice self-control. Self-control begins in the mind. We need to make a conscious decision to monitor our food intake at every meal. In other words—discipline.

Keeping A Diary

Just as the decision to be a healthy individual requires a commitment to good health, the road to a stronger digestion starts with one's attitudes about eating. Clarify your intentions. But, how do you do that? One way is to start a diary. Monitor yourself and your eating habits. Judge for yourself what you are doing that is bad for you. Write it down in a diary. Watch when you do it. Note established patterns. You may be amazed at just how powerful the temptation of food really is. You may even find yourself repeatedly seduced into habits that are self-destructive. Here again, discipline will be your best friend. Reread your diary. Use it to chart your intentions. The solutions will be obvious. Perhaps you have a voracious appetite and consume your food in desperation. Ask yourself, why? Were you deprived of food when you were a child? If that is over now, then is it time to kick the habit? Or perhaps you always finish everything on your plate, no matter how full? Were you trained as a child to always finish your food? Those once seemingly useful strictures may backfire on you today because they no longer apply to your current circumstances.

Your best strategy is to become conscious of what you are eating and to serve yourself smaller portions. Many folks, who are or have felt unloved, compensate for it in their eating habits. You shower yourself with a variety of tantalizing and sumptuous dishes that reward you with the pleasure that makes up for lost love. If these situations are no longer current in your life, you must learn to break these old habits. Discipline to the rescue! Scrutinize yourself using your diary. Study it; then map out your intentions. Even meditate on them or create daily affirmations. These are helpful tools to keep you on target.

Man can survive on one third of his daily food intake. The other two thirds goes to the benefit of the health insurance and medical care industries.

Overconsumption

Overconsumption is the number one cause of indigestion. America as a society epitomizes this. In other countries, traveling Americans are often identified by the size of their stomachs. In USA drug stores, antacids, laxatives, and headache remedies - all needed because of overeating - are the best selling pharmaceuticals. Names like Rolaids, Di-Gel and Tums are synonymous with America. Americans have become an Alka-Seltzer society where the only thing we successfully digest are the advertisements on TV.

The diary method is great for working on discipline and overconsumption and for keeping your weight problem to yourself. But for those who are bold enough, you can go a step further and seek help from your friends. Friends can serve as mentors and support systems. Of course, you can work with professionals, psychiatrists and counselors, but friends have the advantage of being with you when you eat. They see eating habits to which you may be blind. Good friends, if asked in the right way, will sincerely want to help and will not laugh at your request. (Choose the right friend!) Your friend is your eating partner and counselor and can relate to you as a caring observer. You need their third eye just as actors need directors. (For more on *weight,* see p.107.)

Do you stuff your mouth with far more than you can chew? Incomplete chewing results in premature swallowing which initiates a chain reaction of problems. Perhaps you are the type who chews and talks at the same time? This imparts air into the stomach and increases the swallowing of incompletely chewed food. Or perhaps you are a speed eater who consumes whole burgers in a single bite!

Maybe you guzzle down lots of water with every gulp. Whatever your peculiar habits are (we've all got something), let your friend become your mirror. All right, you may lose a friend because of your disgusting habits! But if you have good friends that you want to keep, you will be even more motivated to correct your reckless ways. This method helps externalize your less virtuous habits and eliminates patterns of avoidance and rationalization. You will learn a lot about yourself as well as your dinner manners. Re-learning our relationship to food–what we eat and how we eat it–has a ripple effect throughout our entire behavior and affects our whole lifestyle. Be prepared for positive changes.

FREQUENCY
Second Law of Digestion

*Gluttony is the source of all our infirmities and the
fountain of all our diseases. As a lamp is choked by
a super-abundance of oil, and a fire extinguished by
excess fuel, so is the natural health of the body destroyed by intemperate diet.*
—Nathanial J. Burton

The Schedule

This, the second law of digestion, concerns how you fit eating
into your daily schedule. Many of us never give this any thought. We
eat whenever food is present. This can lead to some rather obvious
problems. The workaholic never slows down to eat a meal. He/she
only "grabs" a meal when "on the run." This is the first step on the
path that ultimately leads to ulcers, heartburn, indigestion, and
other stress related disorders. A workaholic may be so busy, they
put off eating until they are absolutely famished. This wrecks havoc
on their discipline. Food and health are not a priority for the workaholic, which as you might imagine, has many long range consequences. On the other hand, the full-time mother who is always
home and near the kitchen may be tempted to "nosh" all the time.

One of the worst offenses of the "schedule" is eating late at
night. People who do not eat properly during the day end up gorg-
ing themselves at night. If you're a workaholic, this may be the only
time you slow down long enough to enjoy a meal! Or, perhaps you
raid the refrigerator at night? Food eaten late at night sits in the
stomach and often disturbs sleep. It gets poorly digested because
the organs of digestion are in their resting and rejuvenation phase.
Also, the secretion of digestive enzymes is reduced in the horizontal
position. Don't take a nap after you eat. Take a walk!

Some people unintentionally follow an imposed schedule because of the logistics of their daily lives. Their mealtimes may be

fixed to conform to their work schedules or those of family members. These are fortunate events because, regardless of their origins, the effect is to regulate the mealtimes.

The secretion of digestive enzymes is reduced in the horizontal position. Don't take a nap after you eat. Take a walk!

Regularity

The ideal way to eat, however, is to be as regular as possible in both timing and variety of food. Regularity is usually a term reserved for the process of elimination, but regular "in" means regular "out." The planets, the oceans, nature—all operate on rhythms and so does the human body! The individual who wakes at seven o'clock each day, has breakfast at nine, lunch at one, and dinner at six-thirty, is going to have a better functioning digestive system than one whose mealtimes are unstructured. Although most of us do not recognize it, we carry inside us a very influential internal clock that helps us get through the day. You can, with care, reset and adjust this clock. Like Pavlov's dogs, we salivate for food when dinner time comes around. Six p.m. Ding! It's a ritual. The British (traditionally) stop for tea time, the Latins for siesta. Few people choose to ignore mealtimes and that is for the best, because the effect of external schedules has an internal, physiological benefit as well. Your juices start to flow at dinner time and you become hungry. No matter what criticism you may have about the different mealtime traditions, they all have the benefit of enhancing our physical preparedness for digesting a meal.

Eat the Same Repertoire of Foods

Regular consumption of the same foods is very helpful. True, a lot has been said about the benefits of an allergy-free diet that rotates foods. But regular use of the same foods does not prohibit that. It merely enables a diet structured around certain foods whose routine consumption has a regulating effect on your digestive system. Too many invasions by exotic or unusual foods, forces your digestive organs to constantly readapt. Ideally, a diet should be designed in concentric circles with a group of primary foods, in the center, eaten every week and secondary or accessory foods taken along with it. Secondary foods are foods you include in your diet regularly, but are only used in a condiment capacity; for example, miso paste, soy sauce, garlic, salt, olive oil, onions, etc. In a ring around these foods is another group that may be chosen once or twice per month, but are otherwise not regular. Perhaps you include foods like mushrooms or avocados in your diet, but only on an every-other-week basis. Beyond this group lies the culinary twilight zone where unusual and exotic foods (unusual to you) are taken only on special occasions such as restaurants, dinner in other people's homes, weddings, traveling, etc. For example, you may never include artichoke hearts, brussel sprouts, or kiwi fruit on your shopping list, but enjoy these at restaurants and other special occasions.

Please understand: this is not to imply that foods away from the core of your diet can never be eaten, but that "foreign" foods may present some digestive rumblings. Radical shifts in diet can disrupt your whole system and result in sleeplessness, irritability, headaches, fatigue, gas, heartburn, and even colds. On the other hand, being regular in your diet, both in terms of timing and types of foods, creates regularity—an efficiently working digestive machine. Regularity in means regularity out.

Other Cultures

If you examine other cultures you may or may not find better eating habits, but you will find different eating schedules. The Indians (India) eat their largest meal at noon or 1 p.m. and eat only very lightly at 6 p.m. Latin Americans also hold their biggest meal during the midday. The "Siesta" is a mid-afternoon break, usually from 1-3 p.m. This meal is more equivalent to our "dinner," than our lunch. They take their time and eat a lot. Many stores and offices close. Even Western scientists see the virtues of taking the largest meal midday because the largest number of calories are burned at that time and less are stored as fat. The British are famous for their traditional midday break for tea. They schedule their mealtimes early and most restaurants are closed by 10-11 p.m. The French, on the other hand, dine very late and, like Americans, have their largest meal at night. In Paris one can find a full meal even at midnight.

The habits of Indians (India) and Latin Americans are very much in sync with the rhythm of the planets. Both cultures point to the synchronous relationship of the human body and the heavenly bodies. Just as the tides of the ocean come and go on a daily schedule, the digestive fluids in our bodies also follow a natural rhythm. Their ebb and flow is influenced by the cycles of the Sun and Moon just as the menstrual fluids in a woman's body are tuned to the monthly cycle of the moon.

Stop treating your stomach like a compost
and start treating it like a garden.

What are the consequences for someone who refuses to establish a regular eating schedule? If they are young, maybe none. But later, there could be headache, stomach ache, flatulence, distension, or fatigue. Eventually, these problems may become chronic and lead to other problems in other organs and glands. Maldigestion can turn your intestinal tract into a septic tank. Stop treating your stomach like a compost and start treating it like a garden. Establish a dietary rhythm. Keep regular as much as possible. Good digestion yields good health. The inverse is also true—maldigestion creates disease.

Out of Gas!

Perhaps the biggest curse of an ad hoc eater is the loss of digestive power. At any given time, the supply of digestive enzymes is limited. After a meal, this supply is exhausted. Sufficient time must be allocated for the generation of new juices as well as for rest. A meal schedule, structured at 5 and 6 hour intervals, 8 a.m., 1 p.m. and 7 p.m. for example, is ideal. Small snacks of fruits or liquids in between meals will not usually interfere. But heavy meals eaten closely together create an overloading of the system and a backfiring of normal digestion. Food that stays in the intestines too long, or that travels through too slowly, ferments and putrefies affecting overall health and well being. The result is a digestive tract that breeds disease. Instead of an efficient machine, you have a traffic jam where all major arteries in and out are jammed.

EAT CONSCIOUSLY
The Third Law of Digestion

Take care of your intake, physical and mental. Be careful what goes in. Every country has its immigration office...Your body is your country and there are many ports of entry. You should put immigration officers everywhere.
—Swami Satchidananda

Eating consciously does not simply mean the eater should remain awake, even though many people do fall asleep after eating. It simply points to the bad habit we have as a society—that of being disengaged from our bodies while we eat. To say "we eat without thinking" is an understatement. We focus on almost everything else but the food! We eat while we watch TV, read the newspaper, drive the car, ride in a train or plane, talk, walk, work, ride the elevator or subway. Our apologies for this unappetizing mention—but there are those who even eat on their way to the toilet! In accordance with our third law, we can improve our digestion by striving to remain aware of what we eat and how we feel while we eat. Does this sound simple? Maybe, but it is the most violated of all the "digestion laws" under discussion. This law is essentially the gastronomical equivalent of "be here now."

There are several aspects to eating consciously. Perhaps most important of these is the "what, where, and when." We must learn what the right foods to eat are and when and where it is best to eat them. Inconceivable as it may sound, at some time we all find ourselves eating things we do not like. What is that about? Have we lost our senses? Probably not, because we know enough to realize that it is wrong; but we are eating, at least in part, without consciousness. Fortunately, nature gives us sufficient tools to determine what foods are right for us to eat.

The Nose Knows

The first tool of conscious eating is the nose. Many things have been said about this fleshy promontory. It is probably the only sense whose external organ has, for centuries, been maligned, teased, snubbed, powdered, disfigured, refigured, and generally rubbed the wrong way. To say the least, its importance to our health and well being has gone unrequited. But whatever your feelings about its appearance, its function is no less brilliant than its sister senses. Food is to a nose as nectar is to a bee. All it takes is a short walk past a pizza parlor to verify the concept. The nose leads us to the right foods, like the Sirens of ancient Greece seduced its sailors with their sweet songs.

Nevertheless, the art of smelling is shunned by society. Dare you even contemplate bowing your nose to the dinner plate and the aristocracy would sooner chop it off than withstand the affront of a proximal proboscis! Perhaps the nose would be better located on the cuff where it could quickly and discreetly snuff the comestibles. Simply speaking, the nose's primary mission is that of gastronomical reconnaissance. And why not? A little preliminary surveillance is a matter-of-course for other endeavors. Even Boy Scouts probe their paths prior to advancing. Apologies extended to Emily Post for any affront to her blue book of manners: *Etiquette*. But, noses are conveniently located adjacent to the mouth for good reason. When it comes to food—the nose knows.

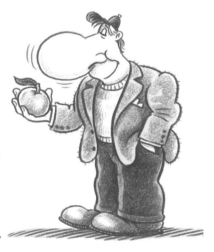

The nose properly proportioned on the body in relation to its gastronomical importance.

Noses will tell us if a food is attractive, repulsive, fresh, spoiled, sweet, heavy, or light. Dining in restaurants does not usually allow us to use our sense of smell prior to ordering. We are forced to select from a written description without the benefit of either sight or smell. (Although some restaurants do flash a display of desserts for your visual seduction.) At the grocers, however, we can see, smell, and feel the prospective edibles. But make sure the grocer does not catch you sniffing! If something is not right to eat, you will know it. Even perfectly fine foods with healthy aromas may respond with a "no" if they are not right for the present time. The nose telegraphs the aromatic essence of a food—made up of its oils and other oxidizing factors—to the nervous system which can either turn on the salivary glands or, in the other extreme, the gag reflex.

When it comes to food—the nose knows.

What A Sight!

Our second line of sensorial apparatus is sight. The sight of food is sometimes the only available method of selection. Still, it provides us with superior information and usually enough to make an qualitative decision. The sight of a bowl of luscious deep blue concord grapes or a colorful salad platter or an apple hanging from its stem is enough to whet the appetite. Your eyes will reward you with many sensational meals. Fresh fruits and vegetables are the easiest foods to choose by sight. Prepared foods, on the other hand, such as baked vegetables, pies, casseroles, soups, quiches, sauces, etc., require smell or taste to help make the right selection.

Taste Tells

Where smelling the subject is not acceptable, and eyeing it is not enough, we are forced to resort to our final instrument of detection—the tongue. Covered with hundreds of tastebuds, this lawn of tonsillar sensors reveals all. Taste offers the broadest range of input of any of the senses from salty to sour, hot to cold, sweet to bitter, mild to spicy, rich to light, and tart to tang. When in doubt, taste it. It is put to best use at home where, in your own kitchen, you can adjust the foods you prepare according to taste. It can make the difference between the sensational enjoyment of a dish or unspoken acquiescence—just another meal. In restaurants, it is usually taboo to shun a dish unloved. But in your home, if something does not taste right, you can turn it down and find alternatives. When you are trying to improve your digestion, eating at home is necessary to provide the greatest flexibility.

Real Hunger

Conscious eating also requires that we know when to eat and when to stop. Ideally, the most digestive energy is available when food is taken at a time of genuine hunger. But eating when truly hungry is the exception in our society—not the rule.

When a farmer has worked many hours in the field, he arrives at the dinner table with an appetite. He is physically hungry. His body has burned lots of calories and after a brief (but important) rest, he is ready to "dig in" to a well deserved meal. You can be sure his meal will be well digested. His digestive system is primed to receive and process it. On the other hand, someone who is not really hungry and eats because the group is eating, brings little enthusiasm and digestive strength to his/her meal. Such a meal is likely to cause some form of indigestion.

No one can teach you to determine when you are hungry. Hunger is part of your instinctual mechanism. You either experience it or not. The problem in modern civilized societies is that the average person never experiences true hunger. Food is always around. We readily succumb to its temptation, fill our stomachs, and rarely, if ever, experience hunger! But, if you pay attention to your sense of hunger and abide by it, your ability to digest and assimilate will increase significantly.

Full of It—Enough Is Enough

Knowing when you are hungry is one thing; knowing when you are full is another. When it comes to our stomachs, we are like babies. Typically, we exceed our capacity only to realize it later after the damage is done. Our minds seem to be on a ten minute delay. Although our stomachs are full, we go on gobbling until we belatedly admit: Oy, am I full!

Holiday mealtimes are notorious for their guests' wobbly exits from the dinner table. They stagger to the nearest sofa where they can repose and sometimes doze. The ancient Romans ate with abandon and regularly regurgitated their excesses. But we are supposed to be civilized and beyond such gluttony. It is just a matter of awareness.

Ideally, you should stop eating when your stomach is half full. This is a discipline which must be self-taught. You can have others help monitor you, but ultimately, it is an individual discipline. We can train ourselves to sense the level of fullness in our stomach. You do not have to be "psychic" to do so. Our stomachs are only 24 inches below our heads—not so far to travel. Do not be discouraged if you fail to sense anything at first. You will improve with each meal. It is just a matter of consciousness.

Eating beyond the point of fullness is overeating. Overeating is finally coming into formal recognition and is being addressed by different groups having meetings and establishing programs. The most famous of these is "Overeaters Anonymous." Here overeating is treated as an addiction just like any other form of compulsive behavior. People who make the effort to join such a group have developed a serious problem which is already at an unmanageable stage. The majority of us suffer from the same affliction, but to a lesser degree, so that the manifestations are more felt than seen.

Chipmunk's Anonymous

A major cause of overeating is the inelegant habit of overfilling the mouth. Many of us tend to use our mouths as a dumpster. We load it up to the max, chewing and frequently talking at the same time. An overfull mouth forces quantities of food down the gullet before it is sufficiently chewed causing, at the least, mild indigestion (dyspepsia) and gas. The emotional co-factor that promotes this type of behavior is deprivation. This type of eater desperately gobbles all. He resembles a chipmunk scurrying around with full cheeks. Over filling the mouth results in incomplete mastication and quickly throws off digestive equilibrium. The solution: take in small amounts and do not add more until the first batch is fully chewed.

Speeding Ticket

Another part of this problem is eating too fast. We all have different rates of eating. Some gulp down whole frankfurters as fast as
a vacuum pump. Others can stretch a cup of tea into a whole meal.
Obviously, one must strike a balance, but the person with the better
assimilation is surely the slow eater. Part of eating consciously is
pacing yourself. If you are guilty of gobbling, then monitor yourself.
Chew more slowly. Make a deliberate attempt to stretch out your
meal and avoid eating at times when you are in a rush. Food rushed
down suffers from incomplete breakdown resulting in flatulence,
distension, poor absorption, vitamin deficiencies, irritable colon,
nervous stomach and laying the groundwork for more complex
problems.

The Value of Saying Grace

One of the best ways to counter this and other bad habits, is to
say grace. Grace is an old world religious and family tradition
wherein thanks is given prior to a meal. This ritual has, for many,
fallen victim to modern times, fast foods, and changing values. You
may say "it's not my religion," or "I'm not religious." But almost all

---

A Sample Grace

*"We are very thankful for all the good food we are about
to eat. We are blessed to share this food with our friends and
family and we remember those friends and family who could
not be with us. We are very grateful for all the good things we
have in our lives. May this food nourish and strengthen our
bodies, purify our minds, and enliven our spirits."*

---

religions have some form of pre-meal ritual—a prayer or a
thanksgiving that does not have to be religious at all. Everyone benefits by spending a few moments before a meal to quiet the mind
and relax the body. Grace aids in the control of bad habits such as
eating too fast, too much, overloading, incomplete mastication, etc.
There does not have to be anything religious about it. It just makes
good sense. You may thank the earth for bringing forth her nour-

ishing foods or thank the people who took part in its preparation. Or, you may thank the universe for allowing you, at this time and place, to nourish your body while others, less fortunate, cannot. If you are really an agnostic, just count to 25 and then start. The goal is to take a small amount of time to focus on the act of eating and relax the body. Take a deep breath...then start.

Time and Place

Time and place are very important for good digestion because eating is part ritual. It demands there be enough time for the "ceremony" else the alternative may be a sour stomach. Too often we eat "on the go" or "grab a bite." If you observe life in a big city, you see people eating on the street, on subway trains, and even in elevators. And how many people do you know who gulp down their breakfast, still chewing going out the door? If you extend the concept of "gulping," its next manifestation is a meal-in-a-tablet, or an all-in-one powdered drink. Don't scoff, such products already exist today!

Ideally, eating is something we do sitting down. But this does not mean in a car or in front of the TV. To eat is to dine and therefore we have "dining rooms" for its full enjoyment. What is your ideal eating environment? How does candlelight, plush carpeting, white dinner napkins, china and Mozart sound? Whether this is your style or not, it is wonderful for digestion. Soft music goes great with a meal as does a peaceful ambiance. Your ideal eating environment, no matter what your style, should have a relaxed atmosphere. Even the family barbecue or picnic is great because the atmosphere is relaxed, with plenty of fresh air (that's good for digestion, see *Deep Breathing*, p.88) and good cheer. Take your stomach out to eat. Treat it like royalty and it will reward you with good feelings and bountiful health.

Silenzio

Some religions practice silence with each meal. This relaxes the whole body and is ideal for focusing on the stomach and the act of eating. Silence affords the ultimate in food consciousness. There are no distractions, no chatter, no animated conversations. You are calm and your thoughts are free to settle on the food and the feelings that come up from it. Alas, most of us are not Yogis or Buddhists and although silence may be helpful and therapeutic, especially for those with bad habits and digestive problems, it is not practical on a regular basis in modern Western societies.

The opposite of silence at the meal is, of course, noise. Sure, everyone talks at their meals, but uncontrolled gabbing will turn any meal into a mess. Talking while eating causes air to be swallowed with the food, creating burping and sometimes hiccups. Loud, boisterous conversation at mealtimes is more widespread

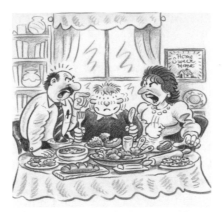

Unpleasantries during mealtime
impact digestion.

than anyone cares to admit. In too many households, mealtime ends up serving as a time for family business, gossip, and the release of anger and frustrations. The dinner table can double as a boxing ring for family arguments and fights. This is how reflux (heartburn), ulcers, nervous stomach and other digestive problems start.

Chew It. Don't Eschew It
One of the benefits of a relaxed, consciously eaten meal is proper chewing. Chewing is the first stage of the digestive process for all solid foods. There are some rules you may have heard about that suggest 60 to 100 chews per mouthful. But most people do not need to make a real count. The aim is simply to masticate the food into a bolus–a fluid mass–before swallowing. No solid pieces should

be allowed to enter the stomach. Counting is good, but a bit puerile for most adults. And if you lose your count, the proponents of this method make you start all over again. Use good sense. Chew your food into the tiniest pieces possible. This creates more surface area on which the stomach acids can act. Large, unmasticated pieces of food entering the stomach cause fermentation, flatulence, and dyspepsia. It takes longer for the stomach to work on the larger pieces of food and they use up more enzymes. The simple, mechanical act of mastication can make a world of difference to your digestion and to assimilation.

Food As Energy

The ultimate aim of our third law, eating consciously, is a kind of spiritual merging with the food we ingest. The goal of "grace," for example, is to bring the food into harmony with you. Although this explanation may sound very "Eastern," it is the basic objective behind the saying of grace. Food, after all, is a form of energy. We consume it to maintain or enhance our energy level. Everything can be defined as a form of energy. All foods, including raw and cooked vegetables, have a pulse which, beyond their vitamins, proteins, and carbohydrates, influence us on a vibrational level.

This effect is not entirely unlike the excitement, calm, or fervor we feel from different pieces of music. Music moves us, we say. Yet, we did not touch it or eat it. Sound does not have a physical form, yet we accept that it can influence. Its vibrational rates are slow and in a range that we can hear. But the vibrations of other things, such as foods, are so high they are beyond the audible range. We can sense them, however, if we train ourselves to feel those frequencies.

You do not need to be a psychic or yogi to sense your food. Most of us have always sensed things but are not conscious of it. The vibrations of different foods blend with our vibrations and influence us by charging, draining, balancing, calming, or irritating us. Think of the last time you felt better or worse after eating a particular food or meal. The vibrational effects of foods are separate and apart from their nutritional content.

This is another reason why grace is so important. It allows you the opportunity to sense your response to the food before you put it in your body. Your response will be either attraction, revulsion, or neutral. In effect, you commune with your food. Whether it is McDonald's or organic grapes, you can harmonize with whatever is on your plate and bring it into your energy field before you touch it. If it is good for you, it will upon its digestion, strengthen, relax or otherwise benefit you.

If you practice, you can learn to use your sixth sense to commune with your food, sense its vibrational effects, and decide to receive that influence or not. If we feel tired and scattered and the food we choose is centering and calming, then we have made a good match. If we feel expansive and the food we choose is energizing, then we will feel more expansive. On the other hand, if we feel enervated and the food is sweet and light, we will feel more enervated. Macrobiotics is a diet that is structured around food as a form of energy. "Yin and Yang" refers to two types of fundamental energies which every food (and every thing) has to different degrees. Followers of Macrobiotics choose foods according to their known vibrational effects. They have charted all foods according to their relative Yin and Yang-ness and have made this admittedly esoteric concept more available to the general public. Yin and yang is an excellent concept to help us manage the "energetic effects" of foods, which makes us more conscious of what we eat.

RULE of SEQUENCE
The Fourth Law of Digestion

I saw few die of hunger.
Of eating, a hundred thousand.
—Benjamin Franklin

After deciding how much to eat and the right time to eat it and focusing in on some of your unconscious and troublesome habits, it is time to turn our attention to the hard reality of the dinner plate and the decisions about what to put on it. Our world of food is vast. The international food distribution system has added new foods and new forms of old foods which, in their attempt to make eating more convenient, has frequently made digestion more difficult. We live in a "gourmet world" where food has integrated with fashion and is more in tune with trends than nourishment. It is getting harder to find basic grains and beans in modern supermarkets and vegetables are more often being imported from great distances, irradiated, and genetically modified. Decisions about what to put on our plates are getting harder and combining the right foods is less obvious with such a multiplicity of choices. But foods can still be ranked and categorized. The order in which you introduce different foods into your system during the course of a meal or series of meals, contributes enormously to successful digestion, absorption, and assimilation.

There are different theories on how to organize a meal and opinions about eating foods in proper sequence are, at the very least, controversial. But any effort to arrange your meal that contributes to the harmonious flow of the different foods through the digestive tract, is the right approach. A well ordered meal permits a smoother handling of your stomach's digestive chores with faster digestive times and better assimilation of nutrients. This means less gas, bloating, heartburn, and similar symptoms and a happier more energetic feeling after the meal is over.

The Order of Eating

Our rule of sequence rests on the theory that the easiest to digest foods should be taken in advance of the more complex foods. An apple, for example, should be allowed to go in first and travel on its merry way without being obstructed by a beef stroganoff or the like. The goal is to keep a steady downward flow of food through the intestines avoiding any traffic jams. Trouble starts when different types of foods, requiring different processing times and different enzymes, clash with foods from other groups.

Sensible Order of Ingestion

- Water and Juices
- Fruits, Smoothies, Soups
- Vegetables
- Beans and Grains
- Meat, Fish, Poultry

This is the plumbing theory of digestion! Although our systems are not as simple as the pipes in your house, the laws of gravity and the mechanics of moving viscous fluids through tubes do apply. Foods can be categorized according to their different densities, water content, and complexity of fats, carbohydrates, and proteins. The denser and more complex a food, the longer will be its journey through the digestive tract and its time until absorption and assimilation. Mixing foods of different categories and different densities complicates digestion and slows the whole system. A digestive tract that is chronically backed up and clogged sets the stage for digestive disorders such as constipation, diarrhea, parasites, and ultimately diseases like colitis, Cohn's, diverticulitis, and colon cancer.

The Mono Diet

The ideal meal in terms of digestion is made up of one food. A breakfast of oranges is one from which you will never burp! Of course, if you eat too many oranges you will violate the law of quantity—that is, you'll max out your enzyme quotient. But generally speaking, digestion of this simple meal will be quick, easy and efficient. Mixing oranges with grapefruits would also digest easily because they are from the same family (fruit) and same subdivision (citrus). Eating these foods is like eating a mono-diet. The same thing can be said for apples and pears. Our stomachs consider these as one food because they are so similar. This is also the case for peaches and plums, cantaloupe and honeydew, raisins and currents, and all the berries.

——— 3 Sequence Samples @ ———

Sample Breakfast
- Juice ⟶ Fruit ⟶ Cereal

Sample Lunch
- Drink ⟶ Fruit, Vegetable, or Salad ⟶ Sandwich, Grain, Bean, Meat, Poultry, Fish

Sample Dinner
- Drink ⟶ Salad ⟶ Main Dish (Grain, Bean, Meat, Poultry, Fish) with Vegetable

———————

Of course, all these foods belong to the larger family of fruits and generally any combination within the same family is considered good. But nature has its exceptions. Each food group differs in taste, texture, nutrition, and thus the way it is treated by our digestive system. Only the pairs we mentioned, those of the same subdivisions, can be considered "excellent" combinations. Salad greens also make excellent combinations. Boston lettuce, bibb, endive, romaine, and green leafy sprouts, are all treated as one food as far as digestion goes. The addition of spinach, parsley, or dill is also excellent because they are in the same class—green leafy vegetables. Again, although all vegetables are good combinations, only those of the same class are considered an excellent combination. Some other examples of same families are a) beans and peas, b) walnuts and pecans, c) sunflower and pumpkin seeds, d) all bean sprouts, and e) all green sprouts.

Liquids

According to this theory, the easiest foods to digest would be liquids. It's obvious that water would be the easiest of anything to digest, but in turn, anything with a high water content would be easy to digest. This means fruit and vegetable juices, light vegetable broths, most soups, etc.

But there are some exceptions. Milk, for example, is a liquid, high in water content, but not easy for many people to digest. It is a concentrated liquid containing lots of fat, protein and carbohydrates. It takes more time to digest because it requires protein and fat digesting enzymes and tends to coat the stomach and neutralize the stomach acid. If you are going to drink milk, do it on an empty stomach, because milk will slow down the digestion of anything taken with it.

Mixing fruits and vegetables is usually taboo. But there are some exceptions: apple, lemon, lime, and tomato are fruits that lend themselves well to mixing with vegetables, especially vegetable juice.

Another problem with milk, and certain other foods, is food allergies. If you have an allergy to milk, it will be hard to digest for that reason alone. The same would apply to citrus fruit if you have a sensitivity to citrus, or to soy milk if you have a sensitivity to soy. Many people have trouble digesting milk because they lack the enzyme 'lactase' which digests the 'lactose' in milk. This enzyme becomes less available as we grow older and some ethnic groups have an inherent lack of it. Soy milk is high in protein and fat and is difficult to digest simply because it is so complex.

Don't be fooled just because something is a liquid. Everything is relative. Yes, soy milk is easier to digest than soybeans, and milk is more digestible than cheese. But if you have sensitivities to these foods, they will be difficult for you in any form. Learn your limits. Test yourself by having only small amounts of these foods if you suspect a problem. Try different brands, dilute them with water, or avoid them completely if there is a problem.

Remember, the liquids easiest to digest are the juices: apple, carrot, spinach, celery, etc. They spend no appreciable time in the stomach and can be enjoyed even by those with weak digestion. Juices go right into the intestines and 95 + percent of their nutrients are able to be absorbed and assimilated by everyone. If you are not digesting your food, get your vitamins from fresh fruit and vegetable juices. Herbal teas are also nutritive and healing, as are vegetable broths. Broths can be homemade or purchased in powdered form and are very nourishing and easy to digest.

Easily Digestible Combinations
Eat These Foods Together

•All Melons	•Green Vegetables	•All Beans and Peas
•All Citrus	•Starchy Vegetables	•All Bean Sprouts
•Apples and Pears	•All Salad Greens	•All Nuts & Seeds
•Peaches & Plums	•Dried Fruits	•Walnuts & Pecans

Purées, Blended Drinks, and Smoothies

Liquids are not always what they seem. A blend of bananas and apple juice does not make banana-apple juice. It makes a purée of bananas. Just because a solid is whipped into a fluid does not make it a juice. You are eating solid food, only in tiny pieces! After all, where does the banana go? This is the difference between blending and juicing. A blender purées or liquefies a solid food. A juicer extracts the water content from a fruit or vegetable and separates it from the pulp. The higher the solid content of a liquid, the harder it is to digest.

One popular milk substitute is almond milk. Almonds are puréed with water or apple juice and then strained. If you do not strain the 'milk,' you will be drinking solid bits of almond. If you use half a cup of almonds to make the milk and you drink it all unstrained, then you are consuming half a cup of almonds. If you have weak digestion, nut milk is an excellent choice, but make sure you strain out as much of the solids as possible. Also, be aware that some strainers pass more solids than others, and some foods do not strain at all, such as cashews, bananas, and papayas. These foods do not have solids that separate from their juice. If you blend cashews for cashew milk (delicious) and pour it through a strainer, the entire contents will eventually pass through the strainer leaving nothing behind. Similarly, bananas and mangos run through a juicer leaving no pulp behind. You are always consuming solids when you juice or strain these foods. Please enjoy them. They are wonderful. But do not be fooled into thinking cashew milk is easier to digest than cashews and do not assume that there is such a thing as mango or papaya juice just because you see it in a store. Read the ingredients and you will see they are purées of the fruit mixed with juice from apple, grape, or other fruits.

Soups

Soups are the most difficult to categorize because there are so many different kinds. There are vast differences between, for example, a broth and a hearty bean soup. Beans are hard to digest and a thick lentil soup is as difficult to digest as eating a plate of beans. Just because it is a semi-fluid does not improve its digestibility. Each soup has to be looked at individually. Some may have a milk, chicken, beef, or vegetable base. They may include additives such as MSG, thickeners, or artificial flavors. Many have flour added, so if you are allergic to wheat, you would have difficulty digesting that soup. The easiest soup to digest is a light vegetable soup or broth. Just chop up your favorite vegetables such as asparagus, spinach or broccoli, add spices, then water, and simmer. Strain off the vegetables and drink the broth. It's easy to digest and super nutritious. Soups, juices, and water are best taken at the beginning of a meal.

Fruits

Fruits are next up on our list of easy to digest foods. Fruits are actually the closest solid foods to water. In fact, their water content can be as high as 90%. This is apparent when eating or juicing a watermelon. After juicing a huge slice, you are left with only a few tablespoons of pulp. Most of the fruit was water! On the other extreme, a banana yields no water—it's all pulp. Bananas are a starchy fruit and unusual as fruits go.

Fruits such as apples, pears, plums, peaches, melons, cherries, berries, and citrus generally spend under an hour in your stomach. Since they are mostly water and soft fiber, no heavy protein or starch digesting enzymes or strong acids are required. Thus, these fruits move through the stomach quickly. But there are exceptions. Bananas, avocados, and coconuts are high in fat, protein, and/or carbohydrates and take longer. Dried fruits such as raisins, figs, dates, etc., are high in fiber and high in sugar. They contain only about 10% water and so differ enormously from fresh fruit. They also spend more time in the stomach—generally 45 minutes to an hour and a half depending on quantity. Fatty fruits and dried fruits are in a league of their own and do not reflect the common attributes of fruits. They belong lower down on our list of digestible foods because they are more complex. But in general, common fruits take between 30 and 60 minutes to pass through the stomach.

Vegetables

Some vegetables digest in as little time as fruits. Tomatoes and cucumbers digest as quickly as fruits. In fact, botanists define them as fruits because they contain seeds, although in common usage they are classed as vegetables. Green leafy vegetables have almost as much water as fruits. A simple salad can take as little as one hour or a little more to digest. Of course, we also have to take the dressing into consideration. The types of salad dressings and how much you use of them can complicate the digestibility of a salad. A pure olive oil and lemon dressing, for example, will extend the digestion time of a salad because the oil coats the leaves making them harder to digest. Tahini dressing or creamy (dairy based) dressings take even longer. Of course, fancy salads like Caesar Salad or Waldorf Salad can have lots of other things in them such as ham, anchovies, croutons, eggs and bacon bits, making these salads more complex. And a bulgur wheat salad includes grains. But in terms of vegetables only, a common green salad with a simple oil and vinegar dressing should take one hour or a little more to digest.

Leafy vegetables are the fastest digesting group in the vegetable family. As the vegetables get starchier, the time required to digest them increases. Broccoli, brussel sprouts, summer squash, asparagus and cauliflower, for example, are so starchy they are usually eaten cooked. This is in contrast to a leafy salad green which would be unthinkable to cook. Steaming broccoli softens the fiber, breaks down the starch, and adds water to the vegetable, making it easier to digest. Of course, the art of cooking requires that you know how long to cook to achieve an easily digestible food while retaining plenty of texture and taste. Less cooking is often better.

Some vegetables can be eaten raw or cooked. Cabbage is frequently served raw in salads and as cole slaw. It has lots of fiber. But it has been known to cause gas for many and thus steamed cabbage is an easier to digest alternative. The whole cabbage family—kale, swiss chard, bok choy, and collard greens, can be steamed for better digestibility, especially if eaten in quantity. Carrots and beets are more fibrous than starchy. They are very high in water content and very juicy, but their fiber can keep you chewing for hours. Because of the fiber, these vegetables take longer than green leafy vegetables to digest.

Potatoes and squashes are the starchiest members of the vegetable family and take approximately two hours to digest when baked. They include sweet potatoes, yams, red potatoes, Idaho's, other tubers like rutabagas, acorn and butternut squash. Most of these are so starchy and concentrated that they should be cooked in order to better digest them. Steamed potatoes are easier to digest than baked potatoes because they are softened by the water. Some people prefer baked potatoes because they does not release nutrients into the water. Foods prepared by deep frying such as french fries are by far the most difficult to digest as well as the most unhealthy. Stir frying is better because the oil does not thoroughly impregnate the food as in deep frying. But steaming or baking is best. Frying adds oils which in itself complicates digestion. But deep frying oil is so denatured that it is beyond the point of digestibility! Fried oils in commercial and fast food restaurants are often used over and over all day long. Once they are heated beyond their smoking point, they become harder to digest and also more dangerous. It is a kind of nuclear meltdown. The molecular structure collapses and welds together in different ways to form aldehydes, peroxides, and acrylamides—all carcinogens.

Some more exotic members of the vegetable family are mushrooms, seaweeds, and sprouts. Mushrooms are high in protein and are considered the "meat" of the vegetable kingdom. One and a half (1½) hours is the average digestion time for shiitake, oyster, and common edible mushrooms. Seaweed is the equivalent of green leafy vegetables grown in the ocean. They are long and leafy and even though they appear black, when you hold them up to the light, their green color is revealed. They come in other colors, too. Dulse, for example, is a hearty red color. But they are all comparable to leafy green vegetables in terms of digestion. Sprouts such as alfalfa, buckwheat, sunflower, clover, radish, and other green leafy sprouts (non-bean sprouts) are also classed in the same family as green leafy vegetables. But because they are so young and have such tender fiber, they digest even faster and are more comparable to fruits than vegetables. Allow approximately one hour for digestion. Generally, nothing in the vegetable kingdom eaten in moderation takes longer than two plus hours to digest.

Beans and Grains

Beans and Grains are the next hardest family of foods to digest. Both are composed predominantly of starch, but are considered respectable protein foods. They even have a fair amount of essential oils. As a group, beans and grains can take between 2½ to 3½ hours to digest depending on the quantity.

Glutinous grains such as wheat, rye, barley, and oats cause some digestive troubles for those who are allergic to gluten. Gluten is the white sticky protein that is responsible for holding bread together. Actually, it is such a good glue that it is the core ingredient of plaster of Paris—wallpaper paste! Whole grains are slightly easier to digest than flour products partly because the gluten is not kneaded as it is in the breadmaking process. Non-glutinous grains such as corn, rice, millet, buckwheat (kasha), amaranth and quinoa are generally easier to digest than the glutinous ones. Of these, millet and buckwheat are the lightest and least concentrated grains and the quickest to digest. Corn causes some allergies and is fairly tough. Amaranth and quinoa are the highest in protein of all grains and fairly easy to digest. Sprouted wheat, which is the most practical grain for sprouting, is easier to digest than regular wheat and has less gluten. Sprouting transforms enough starch in the grain to make it edible raw, albeit only in small quantities. Soft wheat, commonly used in pastries, has less gluten and less protein and is easier to digest than common bread wheat. Sprouted soft wheat is pre-digested enough to eat as a raw snack although, again, in limited quantities. On average, beans take longer to digest than grains. Generally, beans have about 10% more protein. Soybeans can have as much as 40% protein whereas amaranth, quinoa, and wheat only get as high as 20%. This gives beans their reputation as respectable sources of protein, but they are still mostly starch. Peas are the easiest beans (legumes) to digest. When picked fresh or sprouted, they can be eaten raw in reasonable quantities. Lentils, mung, and adzuki can also be eaten raw after sprouting. But chick peas (garbanzos) and soybeans are difficult to digest raw even after sprouting. Although sprouting reduces the cooking time and breaks down the starch and protein, the process is not 100%. You certainly may enjoy these as raw sprouts, but only small amounts are recommended.

Tofu and tempeh are two relatively new foods to American cuisine. Tofu is made from curdled soy milk. It is a lighter product and very versatile. If you have trouble digesting soy, this may be the one soy food you can consume. However, if you are allergic to soy, it would still be a verboten food. Expect about two hours digestion for tofu. Tempeh is a friendly, bacteria-cultured food. The bacteria slightly pre-digest the beans, but it is still a highly concentrated dish and takes 2½ to 3½ hours.

Beans are, of course, notorious for causing gas. This is due to the presence of trypsin inhibitors and complex sugars. Cooking, sprouting, and rinsing the beans reduces these gas causing factors. (For more on *Flatulence and Beans,* see p.69.)

Nuts and Seeds

Nuts and seeds can take longer to digest than grains and beans depending on the quantity consumed. They are definitely more complex than the foods. Some nuts are 45% total fat, 25% protein, 20% carbohydrate, and less than 10% water. As a group, they have more protein and fat (the two most difficult components to digest) than grains and beans. Just rub a few pecans or brazil nuts in your hand to feel their oil. It soon becomes obvious that these concentrated foods must be consumed with respect.

The digestion of nuts and seeds would not be a problem if it were not for commercial processing. In their natural state, all nuts and seeds come with a protective covering—shells. Those hard shells are almost impossible to remove without special nut crackers. From a digestion standpoint, they are signposts declaring: "eater beware." Modern shelling machines remove the shells from almonds, brazil nuts, peanuts, and sunflower seeds with alacrity. The problem is that the convenience of shelled nuts enables us to eat them by the handful. If it were not for automatic shelling, the handful of almonds that we now chow down in three minutes would likely take 15 minutes to consume. Nuts and seeds command (digestive) respect. They were never designed to be eaten in any other way than one at a time. But that's not the end of the story!

Fat, Protein, & Carbohydrate Content of Nuts & Seeds[1]

	Peanuts	Peanut Butter	Pumpkin Seeds	Macadamia Nuts
Water	4.26	1.22	6.92	1.36
Protein	25.09	25.21	24.54	7.91
Fat	47.58	51.03	45.85	75.77
Carbohydrate	20.91	19.28	17.81	13.82
Fiber	8.7	5.9	3.9	8.6

After the invention of automatic nut shellers came nut grinders and with it the advent of a new food—nut butters. Sunflower butter, almond butter, sesame butter, tahini, cashew butter, and of course, the ubiquitous peanut butter. Nut butters combine thousands of nuts or seeds into one jar, making a super-concentrate of this naturally concentrated oil, protein, and carbohydrate food. You can consume dozens of nuts with every spread of your knife. Peanut butter, the most popular offender, has the added complication of not being a true nut. Technically, it is a legume, a pea with a nutty taste. Peanuts are very high in both protein and oil. Just look at all the jars of vegetable oil on the supermarket shelves. Many of them are made from peanuts. Avocados and coconuts, two fruits we discussed earlier, are similar in make up to nuts and seeds and when consumed in equal quantity are equally hard to digest.

The hardest nuts to digest are the ones with the highest percentages of oil, such as macadamia, pine, brazil, pecan, and walnut. Macadamia nuts, which come from Hawaii and Australia, win the prize for the nut with the highest fat content—a whopping 76%.

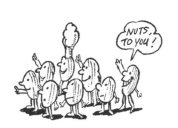

Such high oil content raises another problem–rancidity. Once they are shelled, nuts lose their natural protection from the elements and deteriorate upon exposure to heat, light and air. Sometimes, you can even see it. Sunflower seeds turn from steel gray when fresh, to brown or slightly yellow. The change in color is oxidation, the same process that causes a sliced apple to turn from white to brown. With some nuts, you can detect a bitter aftertaste and others have an unappetizing smell. Not only does oxidation ruin the nuts, it is also harmful to our health. Rancid fats generate free radicals which contribute to aging, break down into peroxides, a component of the plaque that clogs arteries, and aldehydes, which are known carcinogens.

Sprouting plays a very limited role with regard to nuts. Most nuts require germination in the shell and have long gestation periods. Sunflower seeds and peanuts are the easiest to sprout. But even they have drawbacks. (For more details about the sprouting of nuts and seeds, read *Sprouts the Miracle Food,* by this author.)

In short, treat nuts and seeds with respect. Too many will give you a bellyache. When possible, eat them in the shell. They are freshest that way and shells reduce thc temptation of overconsumption. Consume nuts with salads and non-starchy vegetables. When taken in moderation, nuts also combine well with most fruits. Nuts are frequently served with dried fruits which help break up their concentration. Do not eat them with grains or beans or other starches. When nuts are prominent in a full size meal, it will take two to three hours for the stomach to empty.

Despite all these precautions, please do not shun nuts and seeds. They are wonderful sources of protein, essential oils, and minerals. But only if you can digest them! Nature has wrapped them in a hard package because they are so special. You don't need to eat many. Treat nuts with respect and they will deliver high quality nourishment.

Dairy

Milk products are even more complex than nuts and seeds. They contain lots of carbohydrate as well as fat and protein. As mentioned earlier, milk has the particular ability to neutralize stomach acids, slowing down the digestion of everything else you eat with it. When added to a meal, it lengthens the time the meal stays in the stomach.

Protein, Fat, & Carbohydrate Content of Dairy & Eggs[2]

	Eggs	Milk	Cheddar Cheese	Mozzarella Cheese
Water	75.03	87.99	36.75	48.38
Protein	12.44	3.29	24.90	21.60
Fat	9.98	3.34	33.14	24.64
Carbohydrate	1.22	4.66	1.28	2.47
Fiber	0.0	0.0	0.0	0,0

Milk products include a wide range of different foods. The easiest to digest is yoghurt. It is a light, low fat, fermented milk that has been partially pre-digested by the action of friendly bacteria and enzymes. If there is any milk product you can tolerate, it is yoghurt. Other cultured milk products are also relatively easy to digest. They are buttermilk, kefir, sour cream, cottage cheese, farmer cheese, and ricotta. All have a culturing or souring process in common that partly breaks down their protein and carbohydrates. Next in digestibility: soft cheeses. They are easier to digest than hard cheeses because of their high moisture content. Hard cheeses like swiss, cheddar, provolone, parmesan, etc. are highly concentrated in their fat and protein and with a full size meal can hang out in the stomach for three-plus hours.

Other types of milk products can make a difference. Raw milk is unpasteurized and maintains its natural enzymes to aid the digestive process. Although raw milk is easier to digest, it is also harder to obtain. Goat milk products may be an alternative for those who are allergic to cow milk. It contains no casein, a protein found in cow's milk and cheese. Goats are also considered to be

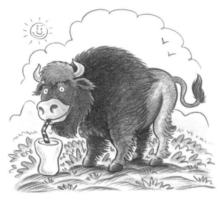

Buffalo milk is hard to digest.
But it's even harder to get!

healthier than cows. They get sick less often, get fed fewer antibiotics, are not usually shot up with hormones. And unlike cows, they rarely get cancer. But, goats produce less milk and therefore goat products are more expensive. Some popular goat milk products include milk, feta cheese, chèvre, yoghurt, cottage cheese, and even goat ice cream.

Other bovines produce milk, too. Once upon a time, buffalo milk and cheese were common. This milk has more protein (3.75%) and twice the fat (6.9%) of cow's milk. If you find some, you will need a strong stomach to digest buffalo milk.

Eggs

Eggs and milk are usually considered in the same category because they are both products of animals. Eggs are also very high in protein, fat, and carbohydrates as are some cheeses, but the proportion of these nutrients in eggs is more suited to human nutrition. Depending on how they are prepared, eggs can take two-plus hours in the stomach. Cooking methods such as soft boiling and poaching make eggs easier to digest. (See *Nutrition Chart For Eggs,* p.35.)

Meat, Fish, Poultry

Fish is probably the easiest to digest of the three flesh foods because of its low fat and low fiber content. Poultry is next and meat is the hardest. Fish can pass through your stomach in less than three hours whereas meats can take three or more hours. These are complex, high protein, high fat, high fiber foods. Their digestion time can be further extended by the addition of other types of proteins or fats such as cheeses. A cheeseburger, for example, with its layer of cheese and bun adds more protein from the cheese and more starch from the bun to the already complicated process of digesting the beef. The more you mix proteins, carbohydrates, and fats, the more complex the meal becomes. For best digestion of an already complex food, have animal foods with vegetables alone and avoid starches and other types of protein. Multiple proteins increase the strain on your enzyme capacity and if you eat too much, can lead to enervation, fatigue, flatulence, and putrefaction.

---

1   Peanuts are Valencia, raw. Pumpkin and Macadamia nuts are raw. Peanut butter is smooth style, without salt. Nutrient Units are in percent. Based on grams per 100 grams of edible portion. U.S. Department of Agriculture, Agricultural Research Service. 2001. USDA Nutrient Database for Standard Reference, Release 14. Nutrient Data Laboratory. www.nal.usda.gov

2   Eggs are poached, milk is whole fat. Peanuts are Valencia, raw. Pumpkin and Macadamia nuts are raw. Peanut butter is smooth style, without salt. Nutrient Units are in percent. Based on grams per 100 grams of edible portion. U.S. Department of Agriculture, Agricultural Research Service. 2001. USDA Nutrient Database for Standard Reference, Release 14. Nutrient Data Laboratory. www.nal.usda.gov

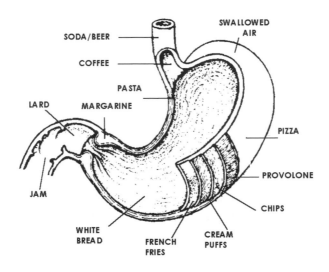

Stop treating your stomach like a compost
and start treating it like a garden.

CHEMISTRY
The Fifth Law of Digestion

*As houses well stored with provisions are likely
to be full of mice, so the bodies of those who eat
much are full of diseases.*
—Diogenes

Everyone thinks that the most important issue in food combining is the chemical makeup of the different foods. However, for most of us, chemistry is at best a difficult subject and the effort to juggle foods according to their chemical composition is too much mental stress for something that is supposed to be a pleasurable activity. The chemistry of foods as they relate to digestion must be evaluated as thoroughly as our other 'laws' of digestion. But to give chemistry top consideration would be a mistake. For most folks, applying the laws of chemistry to our meals is like walking through a maze. One can get increasingly lost and bewildered. Many abandon the whole concept of food combining because of this. Our aim in this chapter is to discuss the chemical guidelines of digestion, but with equal reverence to that of the other laws and guidelines.

The Chemistry of Digesting Protein

Protein has the reputation for being our most important nutrient, but it is overvalued. True, its role in building and repairing cells is indisputable. But its reputation is derived mostly from the mistaken belief that it is required in large quantities and comes only from limited and select sources. Although this is a larger subject that goes beyond our discussion of food combining, we will touch on it briefly. The problem involves three skewed truths or misguided theories: a) we need a minimum number of grams of protein daily determined by our body weight and age; b) protein is only available in a limited number of foods; c) each meal must provide "complete" proteins.

Combining Proteins

This is not a food combining issue. It is a nutritional question and one that has been debated for decades. It was declared or at least popularized by Frances Moore Lappé in her book *Diet for A Small Planet.* She expounded the theory that protein foods had to be combined daily in order to supply the body with the right amount of the various protein components, namely amino acids. Not every-

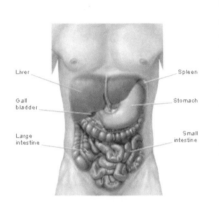

one agreed with her at the time, and in the years since, the almost political controversy she initiated ended with an event, rare in politics or journalism: a retraction. In articles and books she has written since, Lappé has aligned her thinking with the opposite camp–those who believe that combining protein foods on a meal by meal basis is simply an unnecessary effort.

What Are the Protein Foods?

Nuts, seeds, flesh foods (cow, chicken, fish), eggs, and milk are the most well known protein foods. In reality, every food has protein since protein is required for all cell growth. But the relative proportions of protein, starch, and sugar determine whether it is labeled a "protein" food. Soybeans, for example, are considered a protein food—16.5% protein and 10% starch.[1] This is despite the fact that they belong to the bean family which is generally considered starch. Most beans are, like pinto beans—8.21% protein and 25.65% starch. They are predominantly starch foods. Starches and proteins are a difficult food combination to digest, even when nature itself has created the combination. That is one reason why beans should be eaten with respect.

You may be surprised to learn that the highest protein foods are vegetarian. Spirulina and Chlorella, two ancient varieties of algae grown in high altitude lakes, are about 60% protein. Nutritional yeast, a food manufactured by friendly micro-organisms and barley grass powder arc both 35% protein.

Other good protein foods are derived from grains and beans. Tempeh (18.2%) and tofu (8%) protein are both made from soy. Wheat has approximately 15% protein, but the germ holds most of that and when separated from the grain yields more than 23% protein. Wheatgrass powder, made from dried whole leaf grass, is 25% protein. Sea vegetables such as nori, kelp, and dulse are also surprisingly rich in protein, about 25%. Peanuts have about 25% protein (it is part nut, part bean), sunflower seeds 23%, almonds and pistachios 21%, pumpkin (and squash) seeds 24% and pignolia (pine) nuts 31%.

Hydrochloric Acid

All protein foods require an acid medium in the stomach in order to digest. Hydrochloric acid and the enzyme pepsin are the two primary digestive juices responsible for protein digestion. Protein takes a long time to digest. First there is mechanical breakdown by the teeth and the stomach muscles, then chemical breakdown in the stomach and intestines. The protein is actually dissolved by enzymes that break apart the molecular linkages revealing amino acids—the building blocks of protein. Many different enzymes are involved in working on the different links. Amino acids are small enough to pass through the walls of the small intestine and then through capillaries into the bloodstream. The liver receives the amino acids through the portal vein and distributes them to tissues and cells. Your body synthesizes new proteins from the amino acid "pool" to build new cells; make muscles; repair tissue; form new enzymes, hormones, and antibodies. In an emergency, the body can oxidize protein for energy but only as a last resort when the supply of fats and carbohydrates is lacking.

True, if one amino acid is missing, your body may be unable to synthesize a particular protein. This was the issue behind the controversy of protein complementation. This is what Frances Moore Lappé first wrote about and what is meant by the term "limiting" amino acid. Imagine you were making ten peanut butter sandwiches but you ran out of peanut butter after the sixth sandwich. Because the peanut butter was the limiting factor, four people did not eat. In the same way, your body will stop synthesizing protein when one amino acid runs short. That is why a balanced diet with different protein foods is more important than one that concentrates on a particular food however high in protein it may be. Spirulina contains the highest concentration of all protein foods (57.5%), but it is not as good as getting a variety of proteins from different sources. The key is that the amino acid "mix" need not come from one food or from one meal. The liver stores amino acids and distributes them. As long as the general diet contains a mix of protein foods on a daily or weekly basis, your supply is not likely to fall short.

But let's talk about protein digestion. It is best to eat one protein food at a time whether complete or not. Proteins from a group of foods, such as grains, are considered one category. Proteins from beans are another category. It turns out that these two categories happen to mix well. But cheese (dairy) protein, meat protein, and egg and nut protein, each require their own special enzyme brew. Merging them all into one meal would be a prescription for digestive disaster. Mixing several different types of proteins in one meal is just too complex and unnecessary. Too many protein foods exhausts you and your digestive juices. You feel tired, even sleepy. Putrefaction can develop from undigested proteins. For the chronic abuser, this can mean the beginning of colon, liver, skin, and other problems.

Acid and Protein

One might think that acid foods such as citrus fruits would contribute acid for the digestion of protein. However, they can actually limit the production of stomach acid by presenting your system with mixed signals. When protein enters the mouth, the nerve endings on the tongue send signals to the stomach glands to secrete hydrochloric acid and pepsin. But the juices for digesting citrus are not the same as those for digesting proteins such as meat. Although eggs and orange juice are part of the typical American breakfast, they are not good stomach companions. Fruit acids do not activate pepsin. In fact, they may inhibit it.

Starch

Starches are the most common food element in our diet. Starch belongs to the larger family of carbohydrates, which are the most prevalent food category in nature. Carbohydrates are simply a combination of carbon and water. All plants and grasses are carbohydrates. Also included in this family are sugar and cellulose. Starches are very complex with heavy chains of carbohydrate molecules requiring many steps before digestion. They are our best source of fuel for muscular activity. But beware, starches also include so called "junk" food: potato chips, crackers, pretzels, french fries, and so forth.

The first step in starch digestion begins in the mouth with the secretion of saliva. There are three salivary glands: the parotid above the jaw and near the ears; the sublingual below the tongue; and the submaxillary below the jaw. Saliva contains the starch digesting enzyme, amylase. But

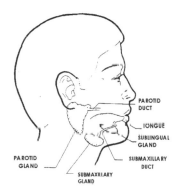

PAROTID DUCT

TONGUE

SUBLINGUAL GLAND

PAROTID GLAND

SUBMAXILLARY DUCT

SUBMAXILLARY GLAND

The Salivary Glands.
Digestion begins in the mouth.

even if it contained no enzymes, it would still be important for lubricating food during mastication. Without saliva, swallowing would be difficult. Saliva also makes the chemicals in food soluble to a point where the taste buds can discern between the fundamental four flavors: bitter, sweet, salty, and sour. Amylase contains the enzyme ptyalin, which begins dissolving the long carbohydrate chains into maltose. Additonal amylase is secreted as necessary in the small intestine until the starch is broken down into grain sugar–maltose. The by-products of maltose, glucose, fructose, or galactose are absorbed into the bloodstream. From there, glucose travels to the liver. The liver acts as a control center dispensing the 'fuel' or storing it as necessary. However, if you are a big starch eater and your body doesn't require the fuel, then the liver will convert the glucose into glycogen for long-term storage or into fat for storage in adipose tissue.

Cellulose

Cellulose is another type of carbohydrate, but an indigestible one. Ironic though it may sound, this indigestible food plays an indispensable role in digestion. Cellulose, hemi-cellulose, lignin, and pectins come from the fibrous portions of vegetables. This may include the skins of fruits, the stalks of vegetables, and the hulls of seeds and grains. Although they are broken by the masticating action of your teeth, and softened by your stomach acids, they are never dissolved. If we could digest cellulose, then we would be able to add a wide selection of plants and grasses to our menu à la cows and horses. For us, the fiber keeps starchy foods moving through our intestinal tract, providing roughage and facilitating the wavelike motion of food through our intestines known as peristalsis.

The Starch Foods

The most common starch foods include:

Wheat	Corn
Rye	Millet
Oats	Yams
Barley	Sweet Potatoes
Kasha	Squashes

Also included are the foods made from these staples:

Breads	Pies
Crackers	Potato Chips
Cookies	Popcorn
Cakes	Corn Chips
Cereals	Baked Potato
Pastas	Mashed Potato
Pretzels	

Squashes, such as acorn, butternut, buttercup, etc., are excellent starches; and vegetables such as cauliflower, broccoli, and brussel sprouts are also starchy, albeit less so. Beans are all starchy even though some have respectable amounts of protein.

This group includes:

Lentil	Kidney
Navy	Adzuki
Black Bean	Garbanzo (Chick Pea)
Green Peas	Limas

As with wheat, foods derived from rice, such as rice crackers, rice cereals, rice cookies, etc., are all starch foods; as are those from other grains such as millet, kasha (buckwheat), oats, and barley. This also includes highly processed (not recommended) foods such as white bread and instant potatoes. Once the vitamins, fibers, and enzymes have been removed, these foods are harder to digest since our bodies must supply the missing nutrients to facilitate digestion. The only thing that is superior about these foods is their shelf life.

Starch and Protein

Starch digestion begins in the mouth with the salivary enzyme ptyalin which envelops the food and continues digestion as it drops into the stomach. The more you chew these foods the better because it increases the surface area on which the enzyme interacts with the food. The big caution, however, is that this enzymatic action stops if a protein food is eaten at the same time. Ptyalin and amylase are both alkaline enzymes that are neutralized by stomach acid. If the starchy foods are eaten first and enough time is allowed for them to pass through the stomach, then the protein foods can be taken without any interference. But if starch and protein foods are combined, then starch digestion will be slowed down until the protein food is digested. The starch then leaves the stomach in a semi-digested state and your system attempts to complete its digestion in the small intestine with additional secretions of amylase. (Amylase is not secreted in the stomach.) Nature also produces starch and protein combinations. A good example is peanuts. They are also difficult to digest, but usually more manageable than our man-made combinations.

Acid and Starch

For similar reasons, acid fruits taken with starch foods inhibit the digestion of the starch. Even one or two teaspoons of vinegar has enough acetic acid to suspend salivary digestion completely. This means tomatoes, berries, grapes, sour apples, and citrus fruits will interfere with starch digestion. There is even some evidence that they not only inhibit ptyalin, but are strong enough to destroy it. If you like orange juice with your toast in the morning, try having the O.J. ten minutes before the bread.

Sugar

Sugar is the simplest type of carbohydrate. It is subdivided into three classifications: monosaccharides, disaccharides, and polysaccharides. Polysaccharides are the most complex form and the least sweet. Starches are considered polysaccharides. Monosaccharides, the simplest form, cannot be broken down any further and are represented by glucose, fructose, and galactose. Honey, milk, and fruit contain monosaccharides. Glucose is the only kind of monosaccharide the body uses. Glucose is also called blood sugar or dextrose. In the liver, fructose (fruit sugar) and galactose, commonly found in milk sugar (see *lactose*, p.26), are converted into glucose for use by the body. Fructose is a main ingredient in table sugar and is sweeter than glucose.

Disaccharides contain two monosaccharides linked together. The most popular disaccharide is sucrose. Sucrose contains glucose and fructose and is the type of sugar in sugar cane, beets, and maple syrup. This is the form of sugar commonly used in commercial foods from candies to soda pop. Too many sucrose foods drain your energy because they use up the B-vitamins and minerals required to dissolve the sucrose link. Lactose, another disaccharide, is the hardest sugar of all to digest because it requires the enzyme lactase, which is abundant in children and scarce in adults. Many people have allergies and indigestion when consuming milk products for this reason. Maltose is a disaccharide that is a by-product from the digestion of starch in grains and is also available in the form of barley malt and rice syrup.

The Conflict of Sugar and Starch

Sugar, whether a monosaccharide or disaccharide, is one of the simplest foods to digest. Even water dissolves it. It requires only vitamins and enzymes and spends very little time in the stomach. Starch spends more time in the stomach; but the problem with combining these two food elements begins in the mouth. As we discussed, starch depends on ptyalin in the saliva to start its digestion. But sugar inhibits the secretion of ptyalin. The signals read by the nerve endings and taste buds on the tongue become confused in the presence of sugar. Thus, even though you chew and mechanically break down your bread or pasta, little or no chemical digestion takes place. The bread has to wait until it gets into the small intestine before amylase can complete the process of starch digestion. This is a bad combination for the sugar food as well, since its passage is slowed down by the presence of the starch food. The longer sugar stays in the stomach, the greater the chance fermentation will take place. Fermentation is the breakdown of sugar into alcohol and carbon dioxide. Carbon dioxide causes gas and distension and alcohol robs the body of B-vitamins.

Sugar also has an inhibiting effect on the secretion of gastric juice. This is why eating sweets before a meal can spoil the appetite.

Protein and Sugar

Fermentation is also the problem with protein and sugar combinations. Again, the sugar foods don't need to spend time in the stomach and when taken alone move along quickly to the small intestine. But protein foods can take hours. Therefore, rather than passing right through on its own time schedule, the fruit or other sugar food has to wait sometimes for a couple of hours while the protein food digests. During this time sugars ferment in the warm, moist environment of the stomach. Ordinarily, the acids in the stomach would prevent fermentation, but sugar also has an inhibiting effect on the secretion of gastric juice. This is why eating sweets before a meal can spoil the appetite. However, if the meal is big enough so that a certain amount of gastric secretion takes place, the subsequent carbon dioxide released will drive stomach acid up the esophagus giving you that warm feeling known as heartburn.

THE SEVEN

P R O T E I N S

NUTS	WHEAT GERM
BREWERS YEAST	BEANS AND PEAS
SOYBEANS, PEANUTS	OLIVES
EGGS, CHEESE	WHEAT & BARLEY GRASS
MEAT, CHICKEN	BLUE-GREEN ALGAE

F A T S

VEGETABLE OILS	ALL NUTS & SEEDS
OLIVES, OLIVE OIL	PECANS, WALNUTS
AVOCADOS	MACADAMIA, BRAZIL NUTS
SESAME SEEDS, TAHINI	PUMPKIN SEEDS
NUT BUTTERS, PEANUTS	SUNFLOWER SEEDS
SOYBEANS	PINE NUTS, PISTACHIOS
FISH, MEATS	ALMONDS, CASHEWS

S A T U R A T E D   F A T S

COCONUTS	PALM KERN OIL
BUTTER	COCONUT OIL
MARGARINE	CREAM (DAIRY)
FATTY MEATS	HARD CHEESES

S U G A R S – S W E E T S

WHITE & BROWN SUGAR	HONEY, MILK
RICE SYRUP	TURBINADO SUGAR
MAPLE SYRUP	BARLEY MALT
MOLASSES	SORGHUM

FOOD GROUPS

S T A R C H E S

ALL GRAINS	POTATOES
BRUSSEL SPROUTS	SQUASHES
PEANUTS	CAULIFLOWER, BROCCOLI
MOST BEANS, PEAS	CARROTS, BEETS

NON - STARCHY VEGETABLES

ALL LETTUCE	BAMBOO SHOOTS
GARLIC, ONION, LEEKS	SCALLIONS, CHIVES
PEPPERS	DANDELION
RADISH	ENDIVE
SPINACH	SWISS CHARD
CUCUMBER	CHINESE CABBAGE
ALL LEAFY SPROUTS	RHUBARB
CABBAGE	CELERY
WATERCRESS	ESCAROLE

Acid Fruits	Sub-Acid Fruits	Sweet Fruits	Melon Fruits
GRAPEFRUIT	APPLES	BANANAS	WATERMELON
LEMON	PEARS	DATES	HONEYDEW
LIME	PEACHES	FIGS	CASABA
ORANGES	PLUMS	RAISINS	CANTALOUPE
PINEAPPLE	APRICOTS	PRUNES	PAPAYA
TOMATO	MANGOS	PAPAYAS	CRENSHAW
SOUR APPLE	ALL BERRIES	CURRENTS	
SOUR GRAPE	CHERRIES	DRIED PEAR	

Fats

Fats are the most difficult of all nutrients to digest and take the longest to move through your system. However, you can help by selecting the finest oils and keeping your overall fat intake in balance with the rest of your diet.

Let's define some terms. Fats are usually thought of as the solid, greasy part of animal foods and oils as the liquid squeezed from nuts, grains, and seeds. The difference is that fats remain solid at room temperature and oils are liquid. Animal fats are mostly saturated while vegetable oils are mostly unsaturated. Both palm and coconut oils, for example, remain solid at room temperature. Saturation means that the molecules in the oil have been filled in with hydrogen atoms; while in unsaturated fats, the molecules remain open. Liquid oils can be made solid through the process of hydrogenation which adds hydrogen atoms artificially. The result is margarine, shortening, and peanut butter (that does not separate). Food manufacturers do this to increase shelf life, make the product creamier, and resist rancidity. Unfortunately, hydrogenated oils are harder to digest. It takes more effort to break down their bonds. Helpful vitamins, minerals, and essential fatty acids are destroyed in the hydrogenation process. Vegetables, grains, nuts, and seeds have the highest proportion of unsaturated oils, as does fish. Chicken and pork have a good amount of saturated fats. Beef has the most.

Do not avoid fats just because the category is hard to digest. Fats are extremely important nutrients. They provide more calories (heat energy) than any other food: nine calories per gram as compared with 4 calories per gram from proteins and carbohydrates. They also help cushion the internal organs, line and protect the central nervous system, feed the skin and hair, insulate us against heat loss, absorb and transport fat soluble vitamins, and regulate fat metabolism. The most important members of the fat family are the polyunsaturates–linoleic, arachidonic, and linolenic (omega 3, 6, and 9). They are known as essential fatty acids because thcy are not manufactured by the body and are necessary for normal cell growth and function. Sunflower, sesame, corn, soybean, flax, safflower, and fish oils are excellent sources. The fat content of your meal determines how slowly food will move through your digestive tract. Fat digestion supersedes protein and carbohydrate digestion since enzymes must first work on the fat in order to separate the different nutrients. Normally, a meal with high fat content can stay in the stomach for three or more hours before it passes to the duodenum. The duodenum is the next section of intestine after the stomach and is the passageway between the stomach and the small intestine. The nerve endings here send signals to the gall bladder to secrete bile. Bile emulsifies fats and starts the secretion of additional enzymes that further digests and separates them from the bile salts. The emulsified fats are now soluble enough to pass through the walls of the small intestine where they are carried by the portal circulation to the liver. The liver combines oils with protein forming lipo-proteins which it distributes to the cells and tissues making, among other things, healthy skin and hair.

In the stomach, fat digestion is assisted by acids, various enzymes, vitamins, minerals, and phospholipids. Phospholipids, such as lecithin, are a natural ingredient of many oil rich foods. They help emulsify fats and are found in every cell and especially in the liver, brain, and nervous system. The more unrefined your oil is, the more likely it contains phospholipids and the valuable fat soluble vitamins A and E. Soybeans are a particularly rich source of phospholipids. Unsaturated oils are easier to digest and absorb than saturated ones and thus it follows that vegetable and fish oils are easier to digest than animal fats. Avoid commercially processed oils as much as possible. They use dyes, caustic solvents, stabilizers, preservatives, and use heat and oxidizers to extract and prepare them. In addition, the oil portion of a plant usually contains the largest percentage of pesticides which are oil soluble. Cottonseed oil is the most common ingredient in low end vegetable oils and cotton is typically treated with more pesticides than vegetable crops. Avoid "cold processed" oils which can involve the use of chemical solvents even though there is no heat. "Unrefined" and "cold pressed" oils are the most nutritious. Remember that high heat turns even the best oils into hard-to-digest denatured foods with carcinogenic by-products that irritate the intestinal walls and interfere with good digestion.

Olive oil and avocados are the best sources of oleic acid with peanut, canola, and sesame oils trailing close behind. Safflower oil is highest in linoleic acid with corn and soybean oils close behind. Other excellent sources of essential fatty acids, and relatively easy to digest, are fish oils, flaxseed oil, almonds, pecans, sunflower seeds, olives, wheat germ, walnuts, and pumpkin seeds. Olive oil and butter have the highest smoking points which means they are the safest for cooking. The smoking point is the point at which the oil breaks down. Butter does not cause cholesterol as was once believed. Only thirty percent of the body's cholesterol is derived from diet. Avocados, butter, soybean oil and the yolk of eggs are all excellent sources of phospholipids. Vegetable oils are not all healthy. Palm kernel oil is a naturally hydrogenated vegetable oil used widely in confections because it creates a thick, creamy texture. Unfortunately, it is not easy to digest. Use of safflower oil is discouraged by practitioners of Ayurvedic medicine who claim it interrupts the assimilation of calcium and creates gallstones. Safflower is also a heavily sprayed commercial crop and, like cottonseed, is not regulated by the Food and Drug Administration (FDA) since like cotton, safflower is not a food.

Oil and Protein or Starch

Oil is similar to milk in that it slows the digestion of everything eaten along with it. It depresses appetite, inhibits stomach motility, and delays gastric secretions. Creams, gravies, butters and oils taken in the same mouthful as nuts, cheeses, eggs, or flesh foods create a multifaceted and extremely complicated meal. The same is true for fats and starch. The digestion of french fries is very slow and difficult because the potato is impregnated with cooked oil. First the oil must be digested before starch digestion can begin. Lemon and green vegetables are about the only foods that are good combinations with oil. Green, chlorophyll rich foods counteract the depressive effects of oils on the digestive process.

---

1   Soybeans used are mature cooked, boiled, and without salt.
     U.S. Department of Agriculture, Agricultural Research Service.
     2001. USDA Nutrient Database for Standard Reference, Release 14. Nutrient Data Laboratory.

CANDIDA, PARASITES
and Flora Imbalance

Symptoms of Candida & Parasites

- Gas & Bloating
- Brain Fog
- Fatigue
- Kidney & Bladder Infections
- Canker Sores
- Vaginal Discharge

- Athlete's Foot
- Ringworm
- Jock Itch
- Diaper Rash
- Arthritis
- Depression
- Allergies

Candida albicans is the term for a group of toxic, yeast-like microorganisms that can inhabit the mouth, throat, intestines, and genital/urinary tract. Yeast live in our intestinal tract all the time. But they are in balance with other bacteria. When the natural flora in the intestines fails to control the candida yeast population, your symptoms develop. After a long-term presence in the intestines, yeast can develop into fungi that actually root themselves into the intestinal walls. The wall then becomes porous creating a *leaky-gut*—a syndrome in which toxins from the yeast enter the bloodstream and weaken the immune system. Candida is also implicated in the bowel diseases Crohn's and Colitis.

Symptoms

The most common symptoms are in the gastro-intestinal tract: constipation, diarrhea, colitis, abdominal pain, gas, distension, and heartburn. But candida can migrate from the rectal area into the vagina causing a yeast infection there (vaginitis). They can also travel through the bloodstream, generating a wide range of problems from athlete's foot to ringworm, jock itch, diaper rash, muscle and joint pain, canker sores, sore throat, tingling sensations, kidney and bladder infections, depression, and even diabetes. These symptoms can co-exist with allergies or aggravate them. According to Dr. Stephen Cooter: "Candida is responsible for flooding the system with an accumulation of toxic acetaldehydes. Acetaldehydes are known to poison tissues—accumulating in the brain, spinal cord, joints, muscles and tissues."[1]

Causes

Bad diet, an out-of-balance intestinal terrain, and weakened immunity are the underlying causes of candida. Overuse of antibiotics destroys the natural flora in the intestines that keep the candida cells in check. Cancer patients undergoing chemotherapy, AIDS patients, infants, diabetics, and others with weakened immune systems are more susceptible to an infection of candida (candidiasis). Corticosteroids and oral contraceptives also upset the balance of intestinal flora. Because yeast mutate, doctors are often forced to prescribe higher and higher dosages of the anti-fungal drug Nyastatin. This makes the yeast stronger and further weakens the immune system.

One of the best ways to test for candida is to eat sweets and observe if your symptoms increase.

Some people have gas for years and feel that nothing helps. They may have developed an imbalance in their intestinal flora leaving a predominance of certain unfriendly bacteria that produce foul odors. This can be caused by any number of pathogenic bacteria, parasites, or yeasts. Candida has become the most famous of this group and regardless of whether it is candida or another pathogen, the symptoms are generally the same. Both the small and large intestine depend upon bacteria, billions and trillions of them, to help in the breakdown and assimilation of food. That is why yoghurt and sauerkraut are good for your digestion—because they contain these beneficial bacteria. But when antibiotic drugs, parasite infection from water or food, or illness disturb this delicate balance, unfriendly bacteria may increase in dominance. They cause gas, foul odors, distension, diarrhea, and constipation. Ultimately, after years of aggravation, it can lead to more serious diseases of the intestinal tract such as leaky gut syndrome, colitis, irritable bowel, ulcers, and colon cancer.

If you suspect you have parasites or candida, consult your naturopath and get a stool analysis. This test identifies the quantity and types of microbes in your intestines and shows how you are digesting your food. *(See Resources)* For anyone with digestive troubles, this test provides vital information and can help uncover more serious intestinal disorders before they become too hard to manage.

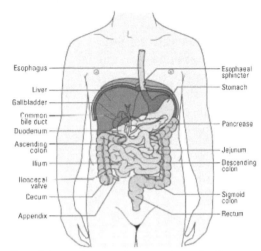

Candida and parasites can invade the entire digestive tract but mostly reside in the small and large intestines.

Use These Techniques to Conquer Candida
- Eat a Sugar-Free Diet
- Take Anti-Microbial Herbs
- Use Quality Probiotics including Bifidus & Acidophilus
- Do Colon Cleansing
- Periodic Fasting
- Get a Stool Test

Anti-Candida, Anti-Parasite Herbs and Other Warriors

- Acidophilus
- Artemisia
- Bentonite
- Black Walnut
- Bifidobacterium
- Caprylic Acid
- Cloves
- Garlic
- Golden Seal

- Grapefruit Seed Extract
- Oregano Oil
- Oregon Grape
- Pantethine
- Pau d'Arco
- Undecylenic Acid
- Wheatgrass
- Wormwood

Four Steps to Clobber Candida and Parasites

- 1. Because candida's toxic byproducts flood your system, cleansing is the crucial first order of business of any anti-candida program. Fasting, colon cleansing, wheatgrass, fresh vegetable juices, plenty of water, detox herbs, exercise, and anything else that furthers detoxification is a must.

- 2. Reduce the yeast population with anti-microbial herbs and phytochemicals. Formulas that include a combination of these powerful herbs are available at your natural food store. Stay on these herbs for only 15 days, then take 5 days off, repeating the 15/5 cycle as long as needed. If you don't take the 5 day sabbatical, the yeast will mutate and develop immunity to the herbs.

- 3. Innoculate yourself with the best "friendly bacteria" (probiotics) you can find. Lactic acid bacteria, especially acidophilus, bulgaricus, and bifidus bifidobacteria, fight back the yeast population and repair the intestinal wall.

- 4. The most important factor in the battle against candida and parasites is diet. These bugs love sugar and simple carbohydrates. The best anti-microbial herbs will not be strong enough to fight your yeast if you keep feeding them. Stop the sweets, now! It does not matter if it is fresh fruit, healthy honey, maple syrup, fruit concentrate, dextrose, maltose, lactose, glucose, sucrose, fructose, or any "ose," —it's all the same to yeast.

Read labels carefully. Sweeteners are pervasive, even in natural foods. Even some rice crackers contain rice syrup. The sweet "un-sugar" herb Stevia will become your new best friend. While you are at it, eliminate commonly allergenic foods such as dairy and wheat (flour products). This diet may be strict, but it is necessary. There are no short cuts. Discipline yourself for a minimum of three months. When your symptoms disappear, you can expand your diet;

but don't fall back into old habits. The yeasts will quickly return. Candida will never be completely eradicated, but your success will be a matter of control—a balanced intestinal terrain, dominated by friendly bacteria, and symptom-free health.

FOODS TO AVOID	FOODS TO EAT
Chocolate	Vegetables
Fruit	Protein Foods
Vinegar	Live Yoghurt Cultures
Wheat	Cranberries
Oats	Sour Apples (Granny Smith)
All Sugars	Acidophilus
Syrups	Whey
Alcohol	Spirulina
Dried Fruits	Chlorella
Fermented Foods	Blue-Green Algae
Glutenous Foods	Millet
Rye	Rice
Barley	Rice Bran
Honeys	Oat Bran
Aged Cheeses	**FOS
*Baker's Yeast	**Fermented Foods

* Nutritional and brewer's yeasts are not harmful. Unlike candida, they do not colonize in the intestines. ** See Glossary.

1 *Beating Chronic Disease,* by Dr. Stephen Cooter, ProMotion Publishing, San Diego, California.

Intestinal Fungus Magnified

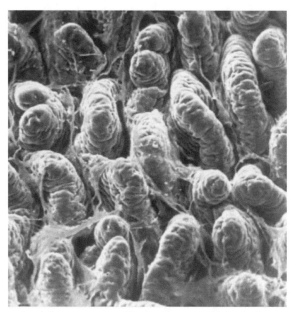

Intestinal fungus magnified a thousand-fold. Over time,
yeast develop into fungi that root themselves into the intestine wall. Anti-microbial herbs and amino acids such as
L-Glutamine and probiotics (friendly bacteria) are used to
weed them out and "re-fertilize" the intestinal terrain.

LEAKY GUT SYNDROME and Inflammatory Bowel Disease

Doctor's used to say: "You haven't moved your bowels in a week or two? Don't worry....so you're a little constipated." But this creates a highly toxic situation that is very dangerous. A healthy person who is eating a high fiber diet should have approximately one bowel movement for each meal.
—Steven M. Rachlin, MD, Gastroenterologist
[1]

If you've been complaining for years of cramps, gas, bloat, diarrhea, constipation, fatigue, and allergies, you may be one of millions of people suffering from inflammatory bowel disease. It is estimated that in the USA alone, one million people have Crohn's Disease (see *Glossary*, p.109) and five hundred thousand have Ulcerative Colitis. Celiac Disease is less known, but nonetheless prevalent. In England up to 10% of the people have "occult" (hidden) Celiac Disease. These conditions result when different areas of the intestinal tract become irritated, inflamed, or breached. Symptoms include constipation, diarrhea, heartburn, nausea, indigestion, gas, bloating, and cramps, and have ramifications outside the digestive tract, causing allergies, anemia, fatigue, weight loss, arthritis, eczema, psoriasis, muscle pain...the list goes on. These symptoms can go on for years with people bouncing from doctor to doctor without ever being properly diagnosed. While these diseases have different names, they have one thing in common—a leaky gut.

The Insidious Leaky Gut Syndrome

A leaky gut is a condition in which the small intestine wall becomes inflamed and breached with tiny pinholes that leak putrid food particles into the blood stream. Your immune system builds antibodies to the proteins in this fecal matter and your body attacks these proteins as if they were foreign germs. That is why it is called an auto-immune disease, because your immune system becomes confused between its own protein and foreign protein. It goes on to attack protein in other parts of the body such as between the joints, causing rheumatoid arthritis. The bone and muscle pain of fibromyalgia and lupus is also attributed to the spread of toxins through a leaky gut. As the cascade of inflammatory reactions spreads to the lungs, it results in asthma. These poisons infiltrate the blood and lymph and overload the liver's ability to detoxify them. Some of this overload empties into the skin, manifesting as psoriasis (itch) or eczema (boils). Other dry skin problems result from the mal-absorption of essential fats and B-vitamins. Anemia and other nutrient deficiencies develop because of the impaired assimilation, in spite of all those supplements you take.

Allergies

The continued avalanche of leaking toxins causes additional chemical sensitivities such as allergies and environmental illness (reactions to common elements such as carpet odors and household detergents). There may be headaches, irritable bowel, gas, distention, alternating bouts of constipation and diarrhea, mental fog, and fatigue. Food allergies are rampant because the intestinal tract is irritated and inflamed. Intestinal permeability compromises our immunity in numerous ways since 60% of our antibodies are produced in the intestinal tract. A weakened immune system makes us more sensitive, creating a vicious cycle.

Friendly Bacteria to the Rescue

The small intestine is approximately 20 feet long and is lined with millions of tiny villi that are like fingers that have the primary responsibility of absorbing nutrients. If you were to flatten out the villi, the small intestine wall would stretch out as wide as a tennis court. This is the enormous surface area devoted to assimilation. Digested food or "chyme" and fiber make up about 60% of the mass that travels through the intestinal tract. The rest of the volume is made up of mucous and bacteria. Ahh, but which kind of bacteria? That has everything to do with your health.

Overgrowth of pathogenic bacteria such as e-coli, salmonella, giardia (food poisoning), shigella (dysentery), or staphylococcus (infection) causes illness. Opportunistic bacteria, parasites, fungi, and candida (yeast), take over whenever the healthy bacteria diminish. Healthy lactic acid bacteria, such as acidophilus and bifidobacterium, must counter the other bacteria. Their dominance is crucial to the strength of our immunity. Before the gut wall can be repaired, the parasite and candida population must be reduced and the resulting toxicity from their overgrowth cleansed. It is not unlike a garden overgrown with weeds. First you must pull the weeds, then you plant good seed and wait, patiently, for the good plants to become dominant.

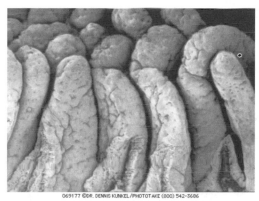

069177 ©DR. DENNIS KUNKEL/PHOTOTAKE (800) 542-3686

The villi under an electronic microscope. Tears at the bottom indicate a leaky gut condition is present.

According to Brenda Watson, a colon hydro-therapist and formulator of a popular candida-parasite treatment program, yeast overgrowth is a silent epidemic.[2] After years of co-existence in our intestines, the yeast mutate into fungi—a plant—that sends down roots into the intestinal wall, making it porous. A majority of leaky gut victims acquire the condition this way. The first task is to reduce the yeast population with antimicrobial herbs. Secondly, seed the intestinal terrain with friendly lactic acid bacteria. Acidophilus is the most popular variety, but formulas that include multiple strains, such as L. casei, L. bulgaricus, L. plantarum , L. salivarius, L. rhamnosus, and S. thermophilus, are preferred. Among them, the bifidobacterium (bifidus, B. longum, B. infantis) are essential to re-pairing the villi. FOS (fructo-oligo-saccharide), a non-digestible saccharide, also feeds and sustains healthy bacterium.

Elimination Diet

Starve your yeast! Even the most formidable antimicrobial herbs or drugs are powerless against yeast, fungi, and parasites if you continue to feed them. They love many foods, but their favorite by far is sugar; not just the white stuff, but maple syrup, honey, bar-ley malt, molasses, fresh and dried fruits. You have to be Sherlock Holmes to find the sugar in foods these days. Read your ingredients carefully; even rice crackers can contain brown rice syrup. Tighten up and get disciplined.

Next, eliminate any foods to which you may be allergic. Aller-genic foods irritate the bowel wall causing inflammation and pre-venting its repair. Chief allergenic foods are dairy and wheat. About 30 million adult Americans and 70% of African and Mediterranean populations have some degree of lactose intolerance. Gluten and its inherent protein, gliadin, are found in wheat, rye, oats, and bar-ley products. Gliadin is so highly allergenic that it is the primary cause of another mal-absorption problem, Celiac Disease. The villi in Celiac patients are collapsed and fail to absorb nutrients.

Supplements & Fiber

Adding fiber to the diet in the form of rice bran, slippery elm bark, or flaxseed is important to keep your food moving through the system and not hanging out and fermenting. Rice bran contains gamma oryzanol which reduces inflammation. Slippery elm is a mu-cilaginous herb that protects the intestinal wall and facilitates heal-ing. Flaxseed is another mucilage that is a bulk laxative, ensuring the regular movement of food through the tract.

The primary nutrient for the repair of the intestinal wall is L-glutamine. Some doctors recommend a dose of 5,000 mg per day to treat leaky gut syndrome. This amino acid is the precursor for N-Acetyl-Glucosamine (NAG), which the body manufactures dur-ing its repair process. NAG can also be supplemented.

Avoid Risk Factors

Two of the major causes of leaky gut and other gastrointestinal disorders are FDA approved drugs—antibiotics and anti-inflammatory drugs. Antibiotics kill all the bacteria in the gut, both the pathogenic and healthy bacteria, leaving an opening for the opportunistic yeasts, fungi, and parasites to move in. Once the latter become dominant, they damage the gut wall and your immune system along with it. Non-steroidal anti-inflammatory drugs, such as aspirin, acetaminophen, and ibuprofen, inflame the intestinal lining

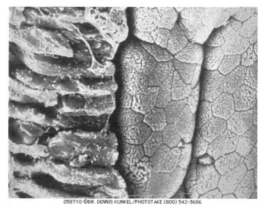

058710 ©DR. DENNIS KUNKEL/PHOTOTAKE (800) 542-3686

Holes in the intestinal wall are visible on the left. This is where undigested nutrients leak into the bloodstream.

causing a widening of the spaces between the cells. Why wouldn't these over-the-counter drugs reduce the inflammation that occurs with leaky gut? Dr. Leo Galland, gastroenterologist and author of Power Healing, explains: "These broad spectrum drugs decrease our production of prostaglandins (hormone-like substances), including the kind of prostaglandins that protect the gut."[3]

Your symptoms, allergies, asthma, arthritis, eczema, psoriasis, chronic fatigue, lupus, fibromyalgia, or failure to gain weight, may take a long time to be diagnosed properly because they don't immediately point to the gastrointestinal tract. Patients often struggle for years before being properly diagnosed. Putting creams on eczema, for example, is like painting a rust spot on your car. It may provide temporary relief, but will return unless you stop the source of the leak. Once on the right program, you can experience significant healing in a week or two. Complete healing may take months depending on the health of the patient and their ability to adhere to the diet program. But Dr. Galland gives us hope:

"The lining of the small bowel changes every three days. It's the fastest growing tissue in the body."

Gut Repair Program

- 1. Detoxify and cleanse the gut using detoxification programs such as colon hydrotherapy, raw juices, fasting, colon cleansing drinks, and herbal teas.

- 2. Kill off parasites and yeasts with herbal anti-microbial formulas.

- 3. Establish a pristine no-risk diet that excludes wheat, sugar, dairy, allergenic foods, fresh and dried fruit, food additives, active yeast, alcohol, anti-inflammatory drugs, and antibiotics.

- 4. Reseed the gut with a variety of healthy bacteria including acidophilus and bifidobacterium and supplement with plant based digestive enzymes until your own digestive strength is restored.

Recipes for Healing Your Gut

Stomach Healer Juice

7 oz	Celery Juice
3 oz	Cabbage Juice
1 clove	Garlic Juice
1 oz	Parsley Juice
1 oz	Aloe Vera Juice
½ oz	Fennel Juice
½ inch	Ginger Root

Use this juice to calm an irritable stomach and soothe inflamed or ulcerated tissues. Garlic is an antimicrobial herb; ginger stimulates the secretion of digestive juices; cabbage and aloe vera are soothing and healing to ulcerated tissues. For ease of juicing, alternate the delicate leafy parsley and fennel with the stiffer celery and cabbage. Make fresh and drink slowly.

Stomach Repair Smoothie

2 tbsp	Wheat or Barley Grass Powder
2 tbsp	Rice Bran
2 tsp	Slippery Elm Powder
2 tsp	L-Glutamine Powder
2 tsp	Bifidus Probiotics Powder
pinch	Stevia
1-2 cups	Pure Water

Grass powder adds chlorophyll, one of the best healers for wounded tissue. Rice bran provides bulk without any risk of gluten allergies. Slippery elm coats and protects the gut wall. L-glutamine is the most important amino acid in the repair of the intestinal wall. Bifidobacterium is the most beneficial bacterium for repairing the gut wall. Stevia is a non-sugar, herbal alternative sweetener. Add enough water to achieve the desired consistency and blend until smooth. Drink on an empty stomach.

1   Rachlin Center for Complementary Medicine, Albertson, NY.
    www.DrRachlin.com

2   Brenda Watson, Renew Life Formulas, available at natural food
    stores. www.renewlife.com

3   Leo Galland, M.D., Foundation for Integrative Medicine, 133 East
    73 Street #308, New York, 10022. www.MDHeal.org

Other Issues
That Influence Digestion

"Gluttony is an emotional escape,
a sign something is eating us." —Peter De Vries,
from *Comfort Me with Apples (1956)*

Water With Meals

Although every issue in food combining raises questions, the issue of drinking water with meals stands out as one of the most controversial. Really, it is quite simple. It is alleged that water dilutes stomach acids and therefore, enzymes, thus prolonging the time in the stomach; or flushes the food out of the stomach before it has been properly treated. Although this is accurate, it is not a simple black and white issue.

Water is an ingredient of many foods and for foods with a high water content, the addition of a modest amount of water is usually harmless. If you have a glass of water after eating a watermelon, for example, it will make little difference. Having water with apples or peaches is not detrimental to their digestion since fruits move through the stomach quickly anyway and do not cause the secretion of hydrochloric acid. Hydrochloric acid will only come into play if there is lots of fiber that must be softened. Certain fruits like coconut and avocado are exceptions. Both contain low moisture, high fat, high protein and in the case of coconut, high fiber.

Salad greens, sprouts and green leafy vegetables of all kinds are all 80 to 90 percent water. Again, drinking some water with these foods does not usually create a problem. High fiber vegetables, however, such as carrots, beets and cabbage, when taken raw, require a certain amount of stomach acid to soften the fiber. This fiber is not digested. Instead, the cellulose acts primarily as roughage. Even in these cases, the drinking of water only mildly affects digestion since it is not a digestible product. Starchier vegetables, such as broccoli, cauliflower and brussel sprouts, have increased their water content during the steaming (cooking) process. You can drink a fair amount of water with these foods as well, although less so than with leafy greens.

Dried fruits are concentrated high fiber, low moisture, high sugar foods. They do require some stomach acid to soften their fruit fiber. But water is also of value here. These fruits are so dry that the addition of water softens them and acts as a lubricant and a solvent. Ideally, one would reconstitute dried fruits before eating. Since this is often not practical, the drinking of water helps reconstitute these fruits in your stomach.

Judicious use of water with a starchy meal helps digestion. But a pint of icy water at a barbeque sabotages digestion by diluting valuable stomach enzymes and acids.

Starchier vegetables such as baked potato also need lubrication. This is usually done through the saliva or by mixture with other foods that have a higher water content. For example, a salad eaten with the potato helps keep the stomach lubricated. A meal of just potatoes and bread would be so dry that you would instinctively want to drink water. A judicious amount of water added here would function as a lubricant to keep the stomach muscles churning and move the food around. The key is allowing for normal motility of the stomach by either adding small amounts of water or mixing your drier, starchier foods with lubricating foods such as vegetables and salads.

Protein and Oil

When a generous amount of water is added to a protein meal, it dilutes the stomach's powerful digestive juices: hydrochloric acid (HCL), rennin, and pepsin. Water and oil rich foods such as cheese and avocados are also problematic. Water and oil do not mix; plus they are usually high in protein. Drinking a bottle of soda pop with your burger both dilutes enzyme capacity and prolongs the length of time the stomach needs for digestion. Too much water taken on top of a full stomach can also act as a flush forcing the stomach to empty its contents prematurely.

Hot and Cold Drinks

Ice cold drinks chill the stomach and slow down digestion by dropping the operating temperature of the stomach and halting stomach secretions. When this occurs, food stays in the stomach longer and extra energy is required to raise the stomach temperature back to normal. The result is an enervation or (inner) exhaustion. Hot drinks also shock the system, although to a lesser extent. The closer the food or drink is to normal stomach temperatures, the less strain on the digestive process.

Flatulence and Beans

Beans have acquired the stigma of being flatulence foods. Gas is produced in beans because of 1) the presence of enzyme inhibitors, and 2) bacteria and fermentation. Beans contain trypsin inhibitors that interfere with the action of trypsin. Trypsin is a digestive enzyme that is formed in the small intestine as a result of two other enzymes, enterokinase and trypsinogen, secreted by the pancreas. Trypsin's job is to break the peptide bonds in proteins, particularly those associated with the amino acids, arginine and lysine.

Beans also contain hard-to-break-down carbohydrates known as oligosaccharides. Oligosaccharides contain two to eight sugars linked together. Raffinose is a trisaccharide containing three links of galactose, glucose, and fructose. Stachyose is a tetrasaccharide (four links) with an additional galactose. Carbohydrates with more than eight links are known as polysaccharides. Their chemical bonds cannot be broken by enzymes in the stomach or small intestine. Instead, the job is accomplished by intestinal bacteria in the colon. Oligosaccharides are also found in grains and seeds and in cabbage family vegetables such as kale, collards, broccoli, brussel sprouts, cauliflower, turnips, rutabagas, and kohlrabi, to name a few.

After these foods pass through the stomach, bacteria in the intestines complete the digestion and in the process produce gaseous by-products such as carbon dioxide, hydrogen sulfide, sulfur dioxide, nitrogen, and methane. Foul odors can be the result of hydrogen sulfide, sulfur dioxide, ammonia, and other noxious gases that are the result of the fermentation of incompletely digested food aging (rotting) in the colon.

Nitrogen and oxygen are the primary constituents of the air we breathe. They are present in flatus simply because some air is swallowed while eating and makes its way through the entire digestive tract before exiting. But swallowed air makes up only a small percentage of the flatulence problem. Intestinal gas is mostly hydrogen, carbon dioxide, and methane.

How to Degas Beans

Enzyme inhibitors are water soluble so rinsing the cooked beans and pouring out the cooking water helps eliminate gas. The same goes for the oligosaccharides. Even frequent water changes is enough to gradually reduce these water soluble components.

- 1) Soak the beans for three hours. Discard the soak water.
- 2) Cook the beans in fresh water for 20-30 minutes. Discard the water.
- 3) If necessary repeat step two until beans are soft.
- 4) Pour out all or most of the cook water, season and serve.

Sprouting beans also transforms the oligosaccharides and breaks down the trypsin inhibitors. The ideal approach would be to sprout the beans first and then proceed with steps 2 to 4 above. Sprouting also reduces the cooking time. Sprouting and rinsing together are the most effective way to maximize bean digestibility. Sprouting alone makes small beans, such as lentils and mung, fully digestible. Beans should be sprouted for 3-5 days and develop a tail that is at least one inch long. Big bean sprouts such as garbanzo, soy, and peas, typically need additional cooking to make them fully digestible. It all depends on the quantity of bean sprouts you consume and how your digestive system responds to the different varieties.

Fermenting foods into sauerkraut (cabbage), tempeh, tamari, and miso (soybeans) creates cultures of active bacteria that also split the oligosaccharide bonds and break down trypsin inhibitors. One commercial product called Beano, contains the enzyme alpha-galactosidase that attacks the oligosaccharides. The enzyme is produced by the fungus aspergillus niger which is present in yeast, soy, and other cultured and yoghurt-like foods.

Other Causes of Gas

Beans are not the only foods that cause gas. Milk and milk products, fiber foods, and certain grains, and imbalances in our intestinal flora are also causes. In milk, the sugar is the culprit. The complex milk sugar lactose is too difficult for many people to digest because adults no longer produce "lactase," the enzyme that digests milk sugar. Undigested lactose often ends up in the colon fermenting and generating flatulence. Cow milk is, after all, meant for cows not humans. Even if you are young and loaded with lactase, cow milk contains protein and fat levels much higher than human milk.

	Buffalo Milk	Cow Milk	Goat Milk	Human Milk
Water	83.39	87.99	87.03	87.50
Protein	3.75	3.29	3.56	1.03
Fat	6.89	3.34	4.14	4.38
Carbohydrate	5.18	4.66	4.45	6.89

Humans are the only species that consume milk after the infant stage. Milk protein also requires the enzyme rennin, secreted by the stomach, to coagulate it. But rennin is absent from the gastric secretions of most adults. The manufacture of hard cheese and other solid milk products increases the digestibility challenge. Goat milk and goat dairy products are much more digestible than cow products because they contain no casein, a sometimes difficult to digest protein found in cow's milk and cheese. If you are a consumer of dairy products, emphasize yoghurt, which is pre-digested by friendly bacteria. Because milk is often a "hidden" ingredient in other products such as desserts, cakes, puddings, cookies, etc., it could be the source of your digestive troubles without your awareness of it. Although lactase supplement tablets are available, they offer only measured symptom relief. The ideal solution would be to leave the milk to cows and babies.

Certain grains such as wheat, oats, fiber, and bran foods are also sometimes responsible for flatulence. Gluten, a difficult-to-digest protein in wheat, is frequently responsible for allergies in sensitive persons. The allergy is an immune response to an undigested protein that acts as a stimulant or antigen. The immune system attempts to destroy the protein, which it interprets as a foreign invader. Your body's response to this irritant can cause changes in the mucous membrane tract from the nose to the anus. Undigested gluten from flour products can also ferment causing gas and distension. Gluten is made up of glutenin and gliadin that form when flour becomes wet. It is so thick that it is used as an ingredient in plaster of Paris and glue. In bread, it is the element that imparts body and firmness. Gluten is also found in rye, oats, and barley, although in smaller amounts. The fiber that comes from the bran of these grains is indigestible. It passes through the digestive tract as bulk. Although it does not cause gas in itself, too much bulk causes a stress in the intestines that can aggravate a flatulence problem.

If you have excessive gas,
check for candida and parasites.

Insufficient hydrochloric acid (HCL) is another cause of flatulence. Some individuals, especially over the age of fifty, do not secrete enough stomach acid to digest their meals. Large pieces of undigested protein and fiber travel into the small intestine and colon where they ferment. Individuals with low HCL should eat smaller, more frequent meals. Food combining laws should be followed strictly. Although HCL and other enzyme supplements help, increasing production naturally is preferable. Deep breathing exercises prior to a meal are helpful. Leg lifts and sit-ups also add tone to the intestinal area. Aerobic exercises are the ultimate solution because they help circulate the blood and the lymph, and enhance oxygen and nutrient delivery to the digestive organs. Fifteen minutes of aerobics, followed by a period of relaxation, deep breathing, and water in that order, is the best approach to increasing digestive strength. If HCL is the "fire in the furnace," then oxygen is necessary to fan the flames.

Charcoal—the Best Temporary Remedy for Gas

The best short-term remedy for flatulence is charcoal. Charcoal tablets are effective, efficient, and non-toxic. Charcoal is nature's premier absorber of gas. It is commonly made from burnt coconut hulls. Tablets are superior to capsules because of their higher potency and purity. They are made of 100% compressed charcoal, eliminating the consumption of gelatin capsules. Charcoal tablets can be hard to find. Ask your druggist or natural food store manager for help. Dosage can be 2 to 6 tablets based on a 600 mg. dose. Start out with the small dosage until you have become familiar with its effects. Although charcoal is completely harmless and beneficial, it will blacken your stool. Don't be alarmed. It is just a benign dye. In fact, it is a great way to determine intestinal transit time (the time it takes for food to enter and depart the body). It may also increase elimination. In addition to absorbing gases, it can also absorb nutrients. So, use it only when needed and on an empty stomach. Take it either in the morning or before bedtime. Avoid eating until one hour afterwards.

Drug store medications for flatulence take a chemical approach. They reduce the size of the gas bubbles so they may pass through the digestive tract more readily. Short term use of the amino acid L-Histidine may be helpful in reducing the sulfur smell of odorous gas and stool. Use of chlorophyll rich supplements such as blue-green algae, spirulina, chlorella, alfalfa, wheatgrass, and fresh greens, also reduces odors, and lines the intestinal tract with this natural antiseptic and purifier. A colon cleansing drink made of flax, psyllium, or chia, taken daily, clears the colon of undigested debris and thus helps keep a short transit time. (For recipe *Colon Cleanser Drink*, see p.92.)

Common Gas Producing or Allergenic Foods

Try eliminating commonly allergenic or gaseous foods. It is unfortunate that beans are included on the list of gaseous foods. They are otherwise one of nature's most perfect foods and our best source of protein without fat. Do include them in your diet. Follow the recommended degassing method *(see p.70)* and enjoy them.

The colon is a two-way membrane that absorbs nutrients and oxygen, but can reabsorb poisons. You may have heard the expression: *the source of all disease begins in the colon.* Good colon health is fundamental to good health. Long term solutions to flatulence involve abstinence of allergenic foods, a close monitoring of the diet, exercise, supplementation, and stress management. Since digestion involves so many essential organs and body processes, the true long-term solution is an overall health improvement and maintenance program.

Common Gas Producing Foods

* Cabbage Family
* Beans
* Milk
* Hard Cheese
* Dried Fruit

* Sweets
* Chocolate
* Wheat
* Onions

How to Stop Heartburn

GERD stands for "gastro-esophageal reflux disease" and it is chronic heartburn—that burning feeling in the center of the chest. Reflux pain in the chest can be so severe, it can even be mistaken for a heart attack. When GERD sufferers want relief, they reach for Tagamet, Zantac, Tagamet, Tums, Maalox, Mylanta, and Rolaids. These are the best selling drugs in the world. Unfortunately, they contain magnesium and aluminum and have many side effects. One heartburn drug, Propulsid, was removed from the market because it caused heart rhythm abnormalities and was implicated in as many as 80 deaths.[1]

Part of the problem with heartburn is that foods are not being digested properly. This can be due to an enzymatic deficiency caused by an imbalance or dysfunction in the pancreas, adrenal glands, or liver. Supplementing with enzymes may improve your symptoms. Conventional medicines can actually compound the problem because they inhibit the activity of hydrochloric acid and pepsin, suppressing the digestion of protein.

Several herbs can help heartburn. *Slippery elm bark* is famous for soothing the irritated and inflamed lining of the stomach or digestive tract. Take it as lozenges or tea. *Ginger* is a proven remedy for all kinds of stomach troubles including colic, flatulence, nausea, and acid indigestion.[2] Drink hot ginger tea or add the fresh ginger to your carrot juice. *Goldenseal* is a tonic and astringent for the mucous membrane lining of the gastrointestinal tract. It helps heal inflamed membranes and soaks up excess stomach acid. Use goldenseal extract or tincture. *Licorice* has a long herbal tradition with scientific backing for reducing inflamed linings and helping sore throat, cough, and gastric and peptic ulcers.[3]

Raw, fresh *cabbage juice* is very soothing to the stomach and can even treat ulcers. *Raw potato juice*, including the skin, can help heal the stomach and esophagus lining, reducing the effects of heartburn. Mix these veggies with carrots, and juice regularly.

Supplements can help. *Calcium carbonate,* in liquid or chewable tablet form taken every two to three hours, is recommended to relieve heartburn. *Gamma oryzanol,* a component of rice bran oil, improves ulcers, gastritis, nausea, abdominal pain, and heartburn. A Japanese study involving patients at 375 hospitals rated gamma oryzanol 90% effective in reducing gastrointestinal distress.[4] Recommended dosage is 300-600 mg daily. *Baking Soda* is famous for neutralizing excess acid. Just mix a teaspoon of baking soda in a glass of warm water and drink at the first sign of heartburn.

Chronic heartburn may be a signal to reformulate one's diet and reduce stress. Reduce excess weight (see *Advice for Overeaters,* p.107) and limit your consumption of foods known to trigger heartburn, such as tomatoes and citrus fruits, high-fat milk, alcoholic beverages, coffee, tea, chocolate, and fried and spicy foods.

The Myth of the Iron Stomach

Our ability to handle difficult to digest foods varies from person to person, and decade (age) to decade. Some people never have stomach problems. They may be active and in good shape or they may be unconcerned with their food or their bodies. They would never read this book. These folks may not worry about their stomachs, but they may have back issues or skin problems or other concerns that are not a worry for you. We are all endowed with certain strengths and weaknesses. The fact that you are even interested in the subject of digestion indicates that this is an area of need. The construction worker who gobbles burgers and soda pop never gives his food a second thought. Of course, he has youth and health on his side.

Unfortunately, there are physical limitations and bad habits do catch up. Look at smoking. The smoking experience is pleasurable. It is only decades later that smoking takes its toll. Although, we have proven that smoking causes lung cancer, we have not yet linked fried foods to colon cancer or artificial sweeteners to cancer. Nevertheless, it is unavoidable—wrong foods and chronic bad eating habits take a toll on our health; if not immediately, then in later years. The guy with the iron stomach may slowly develop headaches, later on high blood pressure, eventually tumors or a stroke. And just because food goes in and out does not mean it has been assimilated. The mechanical process is just about plumbing. But, the chemical breakdown of foods into nutrients and fuel, and their circulation to the cells and tissues, is the true goal of good digestion.

Digestion is more than just plumbing. It is plumbing and electricity. We eat to recharge our batteries, not to drain them. Don't let bad habits sap your energy.

The Peanut Butter and Jelly Sandwich

If you were to follow the laws of chemistry assiduously, a peanut butter and jelly sandwich would be equivalent to a deadly weapon. Here is a food that breaks all the rules. The peanut (protein and fat), bread (starch), jelly (sugar) are all mixed into one. To add to the mess, peanuts are an inherently complex food. The peanut is high in starch, protein, and fat, which makes it difficult enough to digest on its own! Since this popular American food is part of every child's upbringing, we might wonder: how did we ever survive?

The Theory of Relativity

In the world of food combining, most meals break some rules. The question is—to what degree? Even the worst combinations can be properly digested if eaten in small enough amounts. If you have a bite of someone's peanut butter sandwich on an empty stomach, the effect on your stomach will be negligible. And, if there is only a thin layer of peanut butter on your bread, then the bread becomes the dominant food. The stomach digests the bread first and works on the peanut butter later. This is analogous to a lamb in a bull pen. There is no question who is dominant. If there is a lot of peanut butter and a thin slice of bread, the stomach digests the peanut butter and the bread is finished after. Even if there is some fermentation, because the amount of bread is small, it should not cause much discomfort. But if your sandwich has a lot of jam, a lot of peanut butter, and a lot of bread....and you take a big helping, then you have three bulls in the pen butting heads with a lot of rumbling and tumbling. Even if you escape the fight without too much discomfort, the meal is exhausting and everybody is somewhat bruised.

Nature's Own Food Combining

What about nature? She creates many foods like peanuts that are combinations of protein and starch. If nature does it, why should we be so careful with our combinations? Nature does create complex foods. But a peanut is recognized by your stomach as a single food. The stomach digests the starch first and then switches the enzyme secretions to digest the protein. This is very different than having two distinctly different man-made foods that require different timing and enzymes. An example of a man-made food is a cookie. It is one thing to deal with natural grains, but when we grind grains, add sugar, baking soda, chocolate chips, and yeast, we have a man-made food that is several steps more complex than the original grain. From this, the stomach receives conflicting signals, the process becomes extended and ultimately digestion suffers.

Okay, so we all eat less than ideal food combinations....even if we know better. What can we do about it? First, we can hire a censor to work with us. The censor says: Buy the brand of peanut butter without added sugar. Don't eat the fruit that is served with your salad. Leave over the baked potato that is on the plate with your steak. Don't buy cereal with added sugars. Push aside the orange juice that comes with your breakfast muffin. Choose the cookies that are made without nuts, etc. In other words, you can control the degree of clashing foods. When you season your rice, use less butter or oil. If you want to melt cheese on your bread, use only a small slice of cheese. If you want raisins and nuts, mix one-third raisins to two-thirds nuts. If you are at a party and there is a smorgasbord of 15 different foods, concentrate on the vegetables and starches, avoid the fruits and only dabble in the protein dishes. The toughest combinations are the ones with protein and starch, sugar and protein, fat and protein, and multiple types of protein. All these require the production of lots of stomach acid and long transit times. Combinations involving sugars and starches are not as deleterious because the digestive effort is not as extreme. Both of these depend relatively little on the stomach for their digestion. If you eat a bad combination with a fruit, the stress on the system is much less than if you eat a bad combination with a steak.

1   AP Newswire service. Mar. 23, 2000. Washington, DC. "Heartburn Drug Withdrawn: Propulsid Linked to Heart Rhythm Abnormalities"

2   Glatzel, H. Treatment of dyspeptic disorders with spice extracts: Practical use of a new therapeutic principle. Hippokrates. 40(23):916-919, 1969.

3   Cooke, W. M., et al. Metabolic studies of deglycrrhizinised licorice in two patients with gastric ulcers. Digestion. 4:264-268, 1971.
    - Glick, L. Deglycyrrhizinated liquorice in peptic ulcer. The Lancet. 2:817, 1982

4   Arai, T. Effect of gamma-oryzanol on indefinite complaints in the gastrointestinal symptoms in patients with chronic gastritis. Studies on the endocrinological environment. Horumon To Rinsho. 30:271-279, 1982.

THE PERFECT MEAL
A Perfect Day

Sample Menus to Help Make your Meals Work

There is no love sincerer than the love of food.
—George Bernard Shaw (Man and Superman, Act 1)

This is the day you have been waiting for—a day of perfect food combining! Start off with the easiest of all foods to digest—water. You can't get into trouble with water, unless of course it's polluted! Drinking a full glass or two of water is the best way to start your day. It flushes out your stomach and digestive tract and gives you a clean start.

Pre-Breakfast Drink

Next comes what could be your most nutritious meal of the day—a fresh fruit or vegetable juice. Choose your favorite drink of whatever is in season. Carrots, beets, kale, parsley, spinach, and the always seasonal alfalfa sprouts. Or enjoy a fruit drink of fresh squeezed apple, orange, grapefruit, or grapes. You'll be amazed at how much better these taste compared with the bottled variety. Allow at least 15 to 20 minutes for the juice to leave the stomach before introducing solid food.

The Breakfast

Good morning! Today we will be serving brown rice cereal sweetened with rice malt. (Alternatively, you could choose any grain cereal such as oatmeal or grits.) Rice malt is maltose, a disaccharide sugar derived from the digestion of rice. It is only mildly sweet. Certainly, if any sugar is going to be compatible with rice cereal, it is rice syrup. If we chew very well and insalivate the rice thoroughly, we can minimize the inhibiting effect that the sweet malt has on the enzyme ptyalin. Want to add raisins, bananas? Yes, they are delicious, but the more sweets you add, the more you compromise the digestion of the starchy rice. But if you feel up to it, just add a small amount.

Lunch

Now comes the most venerable of all lunch foods—the sandwich. First choose the best bread you can find, preferably from stone ground, organic whole grains with no white flour or aluminum baking powder. (If you are allergic to wheat, choose rice bread or rice cakes.) Next, add lots of sprouts or salad greens, a bit of mustard, a slice of tomato, a pickle, a layer of mayonnaise, add potato chips on the side.....RING! RING! Whoa! Food Combining Alarm!.....that's the conventional recipe. Hold that pickle, tomato, and the mayo. Acid foods like pickles and tomatoes interfere with the digestion of starches like bread. Make a compromise. Since tomato is only mildly acidic, just add one slice of tomato....but perish that pickle! Pickles are cured in vinegar, a very strong acid. Let's assume first that you are buying the best quality brand. Mayonnaise is a protein that contains eggs plus saturated oil and vinegar. The addition of mayonnaise contributes several opposing combinations. If you do not want to give it up, smear on a thin layer. Now for the potato chips. Isn't one starch at a meal enough? Okay, more than one starch is acceptable since starches are not that different or complex. But why must it be potato chips? Chips are deep fried in oil and are largely indigestible since the oil has permeated the potato thoroughly, coating all the starch and prohibiting starch digestion. Nix the potato chips and any other fried foods even if purchased at a health food store. Alternatively, choose baked potato chips or corn chips or even better, slice up potatoes and make your own chips.

Before Dinner Snack

Keep it simple. A fruit, a drink, a smoothie. If you enjoy tea, cinnamon, ginger, and peppermint are all wonderful digestive stimulants to clear the stomach and prepare it for the next meal.

Dinner

This evening's menu starts off with a glass of fruit or vegetable juice followed by a salad of fresh greens and vegetables in season.

There is a vegetarian main course of cubed tofu sauteed in olive oil, tamari, and a touch of sesame oil, with fresh grated ginger, garlic and sauteed snow pea, green peppers, and mung bean sprouts. On the side is a bowl of long grain brown rice. No dessert for now.

A magnificent combination! A vegetable dish with one protein—tofu. Yes, it includes oils and they complicate the meal. But olive oil is one of the most digestible oils and holds up well under cooking because of its high smoking point. A spot of dark sesame oil is added for flavor. Ginger stimulates digestion in addition to adding its distinctive flavor. The vegetables all stand up well under light cooking, adding texture and nutrition. The meal starts off with a juice cleansing the palate at the beginning of the meal when the most liquids ought to be consumed. Salad comes next and in its proper position in the meal, ahead of the heavier foods. The dessert gets passed over.

Just Desserts

There is a time and place for everything. After the meal has had a chance to begin digesting, perhaps one plus hours later, a modest dessert can be added. Before adding dessert, the dinner should have exited the stomach or nearly so. If you pick milk and cookies, you are mixing dairy, a starch and a sugar all in one. If you pick lemon-tofu pie, you have wheat in the crust (starch), tofu (protein), a sweetener (even if it is honey), and an acid fruit (lemon). Most desserts are complicated because they usually involve flour, dairy, and a sweetener. The sweetener slows the digestion of the flour and the dairy slows the digestion of everything. If you chose some fresh or dried fruit instead and had a cup of tea, you would be making a superior food combining decision. But if you choose to have a cookie or a piece of pie, then have it only in small amounts. Take one or two cookies or have a modest slice of pie. You can handle difficult combinations as long as they are in manageable amounts. Remember, the bigger the meal, the less enzymes available for dessert.

THE IMPERFECT MEAL
A Bad Stomach Day

Sample Menus to Help Understand the Difference

The healthy stomach is nothing if it is not conservative. Few radicals have good digestion.
—Samuel Butler [1]

Rise and Shine

Good morning! (Better enjoy it. If you eat like this, you won't feel good for long!) Breakfast today starts out with two eggs; white English muffin toasted; sugar frosted flakes cereal; a glass of O.J. (orange juice—the standard pasteurized kind); and a hot cup of coffee with cream and sugar, please! Sound like a joke? The joke is that breakfasts like this are served in thousands of restaurants across America!

Let's look at it from the food combining perspective. Eggs and toast are a protein and starch combination. The eggs are on a much slower track than the toast and so the toast will hang out longer in the stomach than it ought to. If you used jam, you would have further guaranteed the slow-down on the digestion of the bread by inhibiting its pre-digestion by the enzyme ptyalin in the mouth. Did you sip that orange juice while taking a bite of muffin? Then the citric acid sabotaged the bread's digestion by neutralizing your alkaline enzymes. The acid in the mouth also scrambled the signals telling the stomach to secrete the acids necessary to digest the egg.

Then there is the cereal—an extra, unnecessary food. Since the first part of the meal is already on the fritz, this part is not likely to fair much better. It will only serve to further exhaust your natural supply of enzymes. Even the coffee has problems. 1) It is a liquid at the end of a protein meal, which dilutes vital stomach acids. 2) It is an acid, which confuses stomach acid production. 3) It contains milk, which neutralizes stomach acids and causes allergies in lactose intolerant folks. 4) It is a hot stimulant, which promotes a partial evacuation of the stomach contents before digestion is completed.

Snack Time

It is only 11 a.m. and your stomach is already off to a burpy start. But what is this coming into view? It is that temptress of treats, that babe on wheels, the ever tantalizing office snack cart. There it saunters down the hall parading its bounty of sticky buns, fruited croissants, sugar shellacked pastries, and coffee of every denomination. If you survived breakfast at all, you will need the sugar in this snack for its quick energy and the coffee for stimulation to keep you from nodding off after such an early indulgence.

Lunchtime

More food already? You just had a hefty snack an hour earlier! Well, if you must....Today's special is a bacon, lettuce, and tomato sandwich on white bread with melted American cheese and a cup of coffee. Thanks to the lettuce, there is actually some nutrition in this meal! Also, lettuce combines properly with all the other elements, except the coffee. But the rest of the items do not combine well with each other. Bacon is a protein and a fat and as such conflicts with the bread, a starch. The American cheese is another protein and another fat that further insures the maldigestion of the bread and slows down the digestion of all other foods because it is a milk product as well as a fat. The tomato is relatively innocent in this troop except that its mild acid would slightly interfere with starch digestion in the mouth. Since the bread won't survive the trip anyway, it is insignificant.

Each of these foods also carries an albatross of inherent problems. The American cheese is not virgin cheese but cheese "food" or "processed" cheese made from miscellaneous cheese cuttings that have been recycled. The white bread lacks the vitamins and minerals normal to bread that could aid digestion. They were removed with the germ and the bran. Even the whitish iceberg lettuce, the most nutritious element of this meal, is the least nutritious of the lettuce family and probably contains pesticide residues. Last but not least is the coffee, but we'll leave that discussion for another book!

Pre-Dinner Snack

It's snack time again! How about a bag of salted nuts? Orange colored mini-cheese crackers. Red dyed pistachios? Protein and starch (nuts and crackers) make very poor digestive partners.

Dinner

We'll talk later about why you should not be having this dinner. But alas, dinner is rarely sacrificed; so here goes! First up: an alcoholic beverage—beer or wine. Next, an appetizer of deep fried mozzarella sticks, then house salad, buttered garlic bread, and a main course of Fettuccine Alfredo. Of course, we can't forget dessert—pecan pie with a double espresso, thank you!

Alcohol robs the body of the B-vitamins necessary for digestion and stresses the liver which is needed during digestion. Deep fried anything is unhealthy, but in this case it is mozzarella—a hard cheese, and a fat/protein/dairy product—making it one of the hardest foods to digest. The Fettuccine Alfredo is pasta (starch) with a cream sauce (dairy) typically made from a soft ricotta cheese. Soft cheeses are lower in protein than hard cheeses, but are still high in fat. This dish is very rich and loaded with opposing food combinations. Both the pasta and the cream sauce are equally dominant on the plate and the portions are usually fearsome. Digestion will be compromised and protracted. This is the kind of meal you will need to rest from afterwards, but don't even think of lying down lest you fall asleep! The espresso is more a necessity than a choice. Pecan pie delivers yet another complicated and antagonistic combination—protein and starch in the form of pecans and wheat. To add further injury, pecans are extremely high in fat and the pie is high in sugar. The sugar ferments in the stomach. The pecans prevent the digestion of the pie crust and the oil from the nuts retards the whole process. This is a meal designed for heartburn!

Late Evening Snack

Time for bed, but first how about rewarding our stomachs after such a long day of work? Chocolate chip cookies and milk? Candy bar? Soda? Since food does not digest with the body in a supine position, the likelihood is that much of this snack will lie in the stomach and duodenum most of the night.

Let's accept the fact that food is a material pleasure and eating is a morale booster.

What Went Wrong?

The big problem with this day was not with the stomach—the brain went out to lunch! There are two words to keep in mind to avoid this kind of eating—temperance and abstinence. You don't have to eat just because it's lunchtime. You don't have to take a snack just because everyone else is snacking. Humans are not sheep. Yes, we develop patterns—breakfast at 8, snack at 10:30, lunch at noon, dinner at 6:30, etc. But within those patterns we can make choices—skip the snack, lighten the lunch, give up dairy, cut back on the coffee, etc. etc. Ask yourself the question—Does my stomach feel empty? If not, then perhaps you are eating because you just need a break, a change of pace, some attention. Eating is often a substitute for caressing. We embrace ourselves with a treat. Let's accept the fact that food is a material pleasure and eating is a morale booster.

By piling on meal after snack after meal, you are sabotaging your digestion. Here are the things you should NOT do.

S T O P....

1) Creating a traffic jam in your intestines.
2) Overeating within each meal
3) Eating after 9pm (or within 2 hours of bedtime).

When you overeat or eat two meals or snacks too close together, you risk exhausting your supply of digestive enzymes. By not allowing a rest period to rebuild your capacity, you begin the new meal with a partial supply of digestive juice, setting yourself up for more problems. This is a similar problem to eating late at night. Since your digestive organs secrete less when you are on your back and when you sleep, this gets the next day off to a bad start because the system is still clogged from the previous day. Sometimes you can taste the food in your mouth when you wake in the morning—morning breath. This is from food leftover in your stomach. Not only that, food in the stomach interferes with sleep. If you want to sleep soundly, stop eating at least two or more hours before bed. Your sleep is supposed to be your body's daily opportunity to fast. Your first meal in the morning is your "break-fast." If you get off track eating as in this "imperfect" day, the best solution is to fast and end this vicious cycle. Give your body a chance to rest and catch up.

1   Samuel Butler (1835-1902), English author best known for *The Way of All Flesh* (1903). Quote is from *Samuel Butler's Notebooks* p.90. 1951. Posthumous.

Techniques to Improve Digestion

Man can survive on one third of his daily food intake. The other two thirds only benefits the health insurance and medical care industries.

So far, we have discussed methods of improving digestive efficiency. We have examined the types of foods we eat, watched our chemical combinations, the quantity and frequency of our meals and the time, place, and circumstances surrounding our meals. Now, we shall focus in on what non-food measures we can take to physically strengthen our digestive systems.

Things You Can Do to Improve Digestion

- Aerobic Exercise
- Deep Breathing
- Yoga and Stretching
- Enzyme Supplements
- Fresh Juices & Smoothies

- Appetite Control
- Herbs and Teas
- Colon Cleansing
- Massage
- Sports

Exercise

Just as forest fires need wind as an ally, air increases the firepower in your stomach. The power beyond our digestive systems is "fire." If the concept seems foreign to you, it is because it comes from Eastern philosophy and Chinese medicine. The stomach is the furnace of our bodies. Our food is the wood; digestion is combustion and the energy released is what keeps us healthy and alive. Therefore, anything you can do to increase your "firepower" will aid your digestion.

The kind of exercises that increase oxygen to the lungs and the body are aerobic. These include jogging, running, fast walking, swimming, trampolining, jumping, skipping, hopping, lap swimming, cycling, and dancing. (The best dance for your digestive organs is the twist!) Sports that include these activities, such as football, baseball, tennis, and ice hockey, are also aerobic. Non-aerobic exercises, such as weight lifting or basic yoga, work on muscles and organs, but do not leave you huffing and puffing. Aerobics make a difference in your digestion because they increase your intake of oxygen and its delivery to all your cells. All things being equal, this means that calories are burned better, tissue cleansing is increased, and enzymes are being produced. Most experts agree, that if you exercise one half hour per day, you should see a measurable improvement in your overall health, and that includes your digestive system. On the other hand, if you only exercise one half hour per week, there is not likely to be any noticeable benefit.

Believe it or not, one of the best exercises for digestion is the trampoline. Unlike jogging which pounds away at the skeletal system, trampolining is less "jogging" to the body. When trampolining, all the digestive organs get massaged. The intestines, liver, pancreas, stomach, etc. gently rise and fall without the same shock effect that takes place when your feet hit the pavement. Most of the time our organs and glands oppose gravity whether we stand or lay down. Trampolining enables them to change from their usual positions, free up tensions and release fluids. Hopping on a pogo-stick has a similar benefit, but is less efficient. Swimming is also wonderful. The body constantly changes attitude and pitch and the organs gently flow into new positions. Can't establish a regular exercise program? Walk. Walking after meals keeps the blood circulating and the organs active. Sitting tends to cramp the organs and lying down after a meal tends to turn off or reduce the rate of digestion.

Deep Breathing

If you cannot establish an aerobics exercise program, take a few deep breathes before each meal. Deep breathing brings fresh oxygen to your cells, awakens the nervous system, and sends blood to the brain, lungs, and stomach. Any deep breathing will work as long as you do it for at least 5 minutes; then relax for 2 minutes before you begin eating. Yoga practice includes many breathing exercises known as pranayama. Consult your yoga instructor.

Yoga

Yoga includes many wonderful twisting and stretching positions that have a direct impact on the stomach and intestines. Postures such as the triangle twist, the bow, cobra, stomach lift, bridge, plow, shoulder stand, and other postures, all stretch, stimulate, cleanse, and tone the organs of digestion. In this respect, yoga is an organ massage. Yoga is more than exercise, it's 'innercise!'

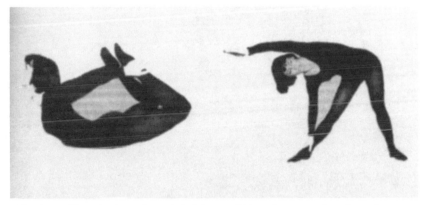

Backward bends, bow, locust, twists, and triangles are only a few of many yoga postures that tone your digestive organs. Consult your yoga instructor.

Massage

Massage is another practice that can be used therapeutically to cleanse and stimulate your organs of digestion. Regular weekly or biweekly massages, using Swedish or other styles, or acupressure (acupuncture without the needles), should concentrate on the digestive system. Therapeutic massage gets blood and lymph flowing, loosens blocks, both physical and emotional/physical and therefore increases your "firepower!" If massage can loosen up stiff muscles, think of what it can do to relieve an overburdened liver or congested intestines.

Herbs

There are several wonderful herbs that are beneficial to digestion. Cinnamon and cloves are stimulants that can be taken before a
meal by chewing on a cinnamon stick or a clove. A drink made from
equal parts of honey and apple cider vinegar, diluted with water to
taste, helps cleanse the stomach and prepare it for a protein meal.
Cayenne pepper is good with a meal to help maintain temperature
and circulation. Ginger root stimulates the salivary glands when
chewed and reduces gas and fermentation when used as a tea.
Cardamon, anise, fennel, celery, and caraway are all good seeds to
chew on after the meal to stimulate the flow of digestive juices, prevent fermentation and cramps, and reduce gas. Charcoal is nature's

Powerful Herbs For The Digestive System		
Charcoal	Caraway	Aloe Vera
Cinnamon	Fennel seed	Gentian root
Celery	Cardamon	Chamomile
Clove	Anise seed	Dandelion
Ginger	Cayenne	Goldenseal
Vinegar/honey	Peppermint	Licorice root

best absorbent of gases for the symptomatic relief of flatulence. It is
made from coconut shells and is completely non-toxic. Licorice is
very soothing and healing to the intestines and deglycyrrhizinated
licorice (DGL) even heals ulcers. Aloe vera is also very healing for
the stomach and intestinal lining and is used for everything from
leaky gut syndrome and colitis to heartburn. Chamomile, while not
a stimulant for digestion, quiets a nervous stomach and is especially
beneficial taken hot, as are the other herbs mentioned here. A combination of bitter herbs such as dandelion, goldenseal, and gentian
root is an old European remedy used to stimulate the appetite when
taken before a meal, and to alleviate indigestion when taken immediately afterwards. Many of these herbs are effective because they
stimulate the flow of bile or hydrochloric acid and enhance the
function of the liver.

Stomach Heater Tea

| 10 | Peppermint Leaves, crushed |
| ¼ inch | Ginger Root, grated |

You can use tea bags of ginger and peppermint, but if you want the best results, make this tea fresh. Crush the leaves of peppermint and steep along with the ginger. Grate about ¼ inch of ginger root into 1–1½ cups of water. Steep for 5+ minutes.

Fresh Squeezed and Pasteurized Juices

Fresh fruit and vegetable juices are nature's medicine chest. You should be juicing regularly for general health, but you can also juice up specific recipes for digestive complaints such as flatulence, heartburn, constipation, dyspepsia (indigestion), nausea, and ulcers, to name a few.[1] Use your juices carefully because they can have different effects. Sweet juices such as carrot juice can stimulate the appetite, but a very sweet juice, such as watermelon, can turn off your appetite. That's why your mother never let you eat candy before dinner! Children who are poor eaters at dinner time, should not be served juice first. Sweet, bottled (pasteurized) juices are rich in sugar and flavor but low in nutrition because many vitamins are destroyed by heat. If you do serve bottled fruit juice, serve it last. Your child's appetite might improve. Green juices such as spinach or wheatgrass can quiet the stomach, but in large amounts can cause nausea. Drink these juices in between meals. (For more stomach and digestion drinks, see *Leaky Gut Syndrome*, p. 65.)

Green Calm

3 oz	Spinach Juice
3 oz	Celery Juice
2 oz	Cabbage Juice
2 oz	Cucumber Juice
1 oz	Green Pepper Juice
1 oz	Alfalfa Sprouts Juice

This calms the entire digestive tract in addition to replenishing vital electrolytes. Best to take on an empty stomach.

Colon Cleanser Drink

1-1½ cups	Pure Water
2 Tbsp	Flaxseed Meal
½	Apple, cut and cored
2 Tbsp	Wheatgrass Powder
1 Tsp	Acidophilus Powder

Digestion is a two way street. In addition to entering, food must also exit! This drink helps maintain regularity. A clear intestinal tract is better prepared to accept more food. Flax is a gelatinous seed and functions as a bulk laxative. This gel-drink moves through the intestinal track like a broom sweeping everything in its path. Follow this drink with plenty of water to keep the mass fluid. Chia and psyllium are also gelatinous seeds and have similar results. Wheatgrass powder is very nutritious and its high chlorophyl content makes it a superb healer for the intestinal lining. Apples are a fabulous source of fiber and are the sweetener for this drink. Green apples are better if minimal sweetness is desired. This drink should have the consistency of a milk shake and will thicken the longer it sits. Drink before it thickens and follow with plenty of water or juice. Take on an empty stomach and eat no sooner than one hour after. Nobody likes a cesspool. So, drink up and keep things moving!

Detox Absorber

2 cups	Pure Water
4 Tbsp	Bentonite Liquid
1 Tsp	Honey or pinch of Stevia powder

This fantastic natural clay absorbs toxic chemical byproducts, quiets the bowel, and slows down elimination in cases of diarrhea. But, it also absorbs good nutrients, too. So take those expensive vitamins and health foods at least 1½ hours before or after this drink. Bentonite is commonly taken on an empty stomach or upon awakening or retiring. Bentonite liquid can be purchased at better health food stores in the colon cleanser section. (See *Resources.*) Stevia or honey improve its clay-like taste.

Digestive Enzyme Supplements

There are many digestive aids on the market that support digestion. The most popular of these is hydrochloric acid. HCL is available in every drug store because it is commonly needed by senior citizens whose production of HCL is reduced after the age of fifty. It exists in two forms, "betaine" HCL, derived from beets and "glutamic" HCL, derived from grains. Some nutritionists believe that betaine is most effective in digesting animal proteins and glutamic is best for grains and vegetable proteins. Whichever HCL you use, it will most likely be accompanied by pepsin, the enzyme that has the primary responsibility for breaking down protein. Pepsin is dependent on HCL because it can only function in an acid environment of 2.0 to 5.5pH. PH is the measure of acidity and has a scale of 1 to 14 where the low numbers are acid and the high ones are alkaline. A pH of 7 is neutral.

Hydrochloric acid destroys harmful bacteria, which is a plus when eating in foreign countries. It has saved many vacationers from the infamous "Montezuma's" revenge. In fact, HCL is our primary defense against food and water bacteria such as salmonella, e-coli, giardia. It is also our best defense against auto-intoxication. This occurs when incompletely digested food rots inside our intestinal tract spreading their toxic byproducts into our system and initiating a wide variety of chronic illnesses if it remains unchecked.

When the hydrochloric acid content of the gastric fluid is deficient or absent, grave results must gradually and inevitably appear in the human metabolism. First of all, we shall have an increasing and gradual starvation of the mineral elements in the food supply. The food will be incompletely digested and failure of assimilation must occur. Secondly, a septic process (pus forming toxins in the blood or tissues) of the tissues will appear; pyorrhea, dyspepsia, nephritis, appendicitis, boils, abscesses, pneumonia, etc., will become increasingly manifest. Again, a normal gastric fluid demands activity of the gall bladder contents and the pancreas for neutralization. Deficiency of normal acid leads to stagnation of these organs, causing diabetes and gallstones. In other words, an absence or a great deficiency of HCL gives rise to multitudinous degenerative reactions and prepares the way for all forms of degenerative disease.[2]

A good digestive enzyme supplement used judiciously can also restimulate natural production of HCL. Potassium and ammonium chloride aid in acidifying the intestinal tract and getting at the cause of the lack of HCL. These two minerals control chloride ion concentrations and regulate intestinal function.

If you walk into a pharmacy in America, you will notice the longest aisle is the one with remedies for acid indigestion. Over acidity is an epidemic complaint. Ironically, it is often caused by a lack of hydrochloric acid. When there is insufficient HCL, protein foods can putrefy releasing unhealthful fermentation acids. These by-products, if repeated over time, can cause a wide range of problems from ulcers to colon cancer. Taking antacid tablets or liquids, as people often do, neutralizes the acids of fermentation, but makes the stomach too alkaline for the normal digestion of food.

Primary Digestive Enzymes

• Lipase	• Amylase	• Phytase
• Sucrase	• Bile	• Bromelain
• Lactase	• Pancreatin	• Betaine HCL
• Cellulase	• Protease	• Glutamic HCL
• Pepsin		• Papain

Common Digestive Supplements

Non-HCL digestive supplements contain other enzymes that serve different aspects of the digestive process. The papaya fruit has long had a reputation for its protein (proteolytic) digesting enzyme, papain. Papain is found in the unripe papaya fruit and leaves. Natives who live in the subtropics where papaya is abundant, use the leaves as a meat tenderizer. They slit the leaves to allow the milky juice to ooze and then wrap the meat in them. The papain in the juice partially digests the meat thereby increasing its tenderness. Papain also helps digest the factor in gluten (gliadin) that affects persons with Celiac Disease. These people cannot tolerate wheat or other glutenous grains. Bromelain, derived from pineapples, is another tropical fruit enzyme that breaks proteins apart into amino acids. Medical doctors have also used bromelain to clean out arteries and reduce inflammation; it stimulates the body's production of the anti-Cancer compounds Interleukin 1, Interleukin 6, and Tumor Necrosis Factor (TNF).

Fats are digested by lipase and bile. The latter is often derived from oxen and would not be acceptable to vegetarians. Fat digesting enzymes can improve constipation by stimulating the flow of bile and improving the efficiency of the gall bladder.

Protein is digested by protease, trypsin, HCL, and pancreatin. The pancreas secretes a range of enzymes called pancreatin that work on protein, starch, cholesterol, RNA, and DNA. Pancreatin also prevents the proliferation of detrimental microorganisms such as parasites. All proteases, or protein digestive enzymes, split proteins into peptides and amino acids.

Amylase is also secreted by the pancreas, but is first provided by the salivary glands and has the primary responsibility for the digestion of starch. Starches are carbohydrates that include sugar. Many sugars have their own specific enzymes. Sucrose, lactose, and maltose, for example, are digested by the enzymes sucrase, lactase, and maltase. Fiber, on the other hand, is a complex carbohydrate with so many chemical links (polysaccharides) that it is virtually indigestible. Cellulose is the most ubiquitous carbohydrate in nature and it is non-digestible. Its very important function is simply to contribute bulk to move the intestinal contents along on their journey.

The Role of Enzyme Supplements

Digestive aids help reclaim digestive strength whenever the digestive system is weak. When used in this fashion, they are a bridge to help you get back on your feet. Some people's digestion is so weak that they depend on them on a regular basis. If routine use is necessary, choose plant based enzymes (phytase, sucrase, maltase, protease, amylase, lipase, etc.) instead of HCL and pancreatic juice. Plant based enzymes work in the broadest range of pH environments. Every raw fruit or vegetable delivers an array of plant enzymes that assist in its digestion. Diets high in cooked vegetables, fried foods, canned, and frozen foods are lacking in enzymes and can benefit from supplementation. Enzymes perform many functions in the body including the repair and removal of old or diseased tissue. The main argument against exogenous enzymes (from supplements) is that they create a lethargy in our own enzyme-producing organs. If this is true, then supplements, in particular animal derived enzymes, should be used under the guidance of a health professional or on a limited use basis.

*The ultimate challenge is to stop eating before you
are full. It may sound too good to be true,
but with this simple act alone,
all of your digestive troubles could be solved.*

Secrets to Controlling Your Appetite

Controlling how much you eat is one of the keys to good digestion. Of course you could discipline yourself by preparing your plate with a pre-determined, fixed amount of food or by simply not taking a second helping. But the ultimate challenge is to stop eating before you are full. It may sound too good to be true, but with this simple act alone, all of your digestive troubles could be solved. Another trick is to get up from the table and just walk away. Even better, brush your teeth. You simply won't go back to eating again. It works every time.

Certain foods also control appetite. Concentrated green juices such as wheatgrass, barley grass, chlorella, spinach, and parsley seem to neutralize appetite. Their concentrated nutrition and protein may possibly create a satiety. Psyllium, flax, and chia seeds develop a mucilage when blended with water or juice. This drink creates a feeling of fullness due to its high bulk fiber, which is wonderful for intestinal cleansing. If you have a problem controlling your appetite, "drink" green or make a flax seed smoothie. (See recipe *Colon Cleanser Drink,* p. 92.)

Factors That Weaken Digestion

Sometimes it seems that everything we do has an impact on digestion. It is affected by how, where, and when we eat; our mood; our company....even taking aspirin affects it. If you are trying to optimize your digestion, here are some considerations for you to keep in mind.

Avoid Eating While...

* Walking
* Watching TV
* Standing
* Driving

* Talking on the telephone
* Reading the newspaper
* Riding in an elevator
* Lying

We take the act of eating so much for granted that we rarely pay attention to it. When reading the newspaper, most people finish eating when they finish reading. If munching when on the phone, they stop munching upon hanging up. The talking or reading is the overriding activity...not the eating. Talking also forces air to be swallowed with the food and usually shortens the degree of mastication. Walking is a wonderful activity to stimulate digestion after a meal, but not during a meal. Food should be eaten sitting down.

Stop Taking Antibiotics and Aspirin

Antibiotics kill all the bacteria in the gut, both good and bad, which throws the intestinal terrain into a free-for-all where opportunistic yeasts, fungi, and parasites can move in and destroy normal digestion. Aspirin, acetaminophen, and ibuprofen, are all non-steroidal, anti-inflammatory drugs, which inflame the intestinal lining causing inflammatory bowel disease. (See *Leaky Gut Syndrome*, p.59, 63.)

Parties

Food is entertainment and entertainers usually provide food. But that does not give you license to lose all your discipline at a party. Just because pretzels and potato chips are party standards does not mean there are no healthier alternatives. Use the party as an opportunity to introduce your friends to new and healthier foods. New food ideas and tastes make your party more interesting. Your guests will be impressed and they will have something to talk about. In this way, your friends will start to support your effort to eat better and learn something in the process.

The Conundrum of the Business Lunch

By the same token, food should not be a tool of business—unless you are in the food business! Business needs your attention and if we have been saying anything in this book, it is that when you are eating, your body needs your attention. So don't put yourself into a compromising position. Business is not always good for digestion. Stress over money or tension about a deal can turn a healthy stomach sour. Make your deal first, then relax and enjoy your meal.

The Six O'Clock Fight

For many families, mealtime is often the only opportunity they have to convene during the day. Consequently, it is often devoted to family "business" and this can lead to discussion or disagreement. In this atmosphere, it is not unheard of to underscore your argument with some flying spaghetti. Or you may cool down your adversary with some soda pop. In either case, digestion suffers. Anger tightens the ducts and glands and reduces the secretion of hormones, enzymes, and digestive juices. The nervous system, which is in charge of sending the proper signals to the organs of digestion, is overridden by the emotions of the moment. You will literally lose your appetite and turn off your stomach. On the other hand, good company and stimulating conversation are the most supportive conditions for good digestion. (See *Time and Place*, p.19.)

One should eat to live, not live to eat.—Moliére[3]

A Happy Eater Digests Best

It may sound facetious, but you can eat the same meal and have completely different results depending on your mood. A perfect food combined meal eaten when depressed can rot in your stomach. However, a gluttonous feast can turn out well if there is a positive attitude, good company, and good cheer. So, consider your mood when you eat and be happy. (For more on *emotions and digestion*, see *Swami Digestanada*, p.103.)

*The body and the mind are interconnected and
interdependent. The body expresses
the thoughts of the mind. Constantly thinking
crooked thoughts will create a crooked body.
If you have a happy mind, your face and body will
reflect that happiness. Everybody will know
something beautiful is happening within you.*

—Swami Satchidananda[4]

1   For recipes about specific complaints read *Power Juices Super Drinks, Quick and Delicious Recipes to Prevent and Reverse Disease* by this author (Steve Meyerowitz). 454 pgs. Kensington Publishing, New York. 2000.

2   From Professor A.E. Austin, in his book the *Manual of Clinical Chemistry.*

3   *"One should eat to live, not live to eat."* –Molière (1622-73), French dramatist. Spoken by Valère, in *The Miser*, act 3, sc. 1.

4   From *Beyond Words.* by Swami Satchidananda. Holt, Reinhart and Winston, New York. 1977.

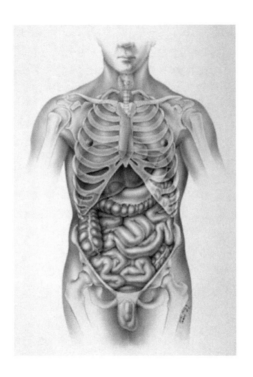

The road to health is paved
with good intestines.

Digestive Wisdom

Interview by the Author with

Swami Digestananda

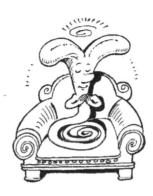

Guru of the Gut

Swami Digestananda is widely known as the "guru of the gut." He is thought to be the originator of the food combining theory, and is the supreme authority of all things gastronomical. Here, he shares his splendiferous wisdom on the subject of digestion received by postless transmission from his retreat high atop Mount Metamucil in the Herralayas.

Dear Swami, tell us about your diet.

I have tried every possible diet. I have been a vegetarian for more than 90 years; I was a strict raw foodist for 40 years; a macrobiotic for 25 years, and a fruitarian for 12 years. During my stay in the United States, I became an ice-creamarian.

You ate ice cream?

Yes. You see, ice cream is a happy food. People eat it because it makes them feel good. Sometimes they don't feel so good, if they eat too much, or if they are allergic, but generally, eating ice cream makes people happy. Since I am in the business of teaching people to find their inner joy, I sought the secrets of this milky miracle. Why is it this food makes so many people happy? Is it special vitamins? Is it the pretty colors? Is it the hormones from the holy cow?

What did you learn?

First of all, I learned that there are many different kinds of ice creams. I don't mean the flavors or the colors, but the basic concept and purpose of it. I learned that on an ice cream diet, one would be best suited to live in America, preferably Disneyland. Here in Tibet, we have only two flavors of ice cream, cow and goat. But in America, you have Baskin and Robbins. I could eat all day at Baskin and Robbins. Then, I would go and eat at Ben & Jerry's. That was an entirely different experience. But there, I learned about the Rainforest, third world commerce, and Vermont, all thanks to the ice cream. Only in America is ice cream a whole meal. You can have ice cream sandwiches, ice cream cookies, ice cream with nuts, sprinkles, M&M's, and frozen yoghurt. I knew I was breaking my diet, but at least everything was vegetarian.

Did it make you happy?

Yes, in addition to some indigestion. Ice cream appears to have the capacity to tickle your insides. But it has nothing to do with the ingredients. I believe ice cream puts you into an altered state. When you eat it, you think you are being given a treat. In truth, ice cream has no power itself. It is neither good nor evil. Food, in general, has no morality. You may feel sinful when you eat devil's food cake, but there are no devils around it nor are there angels around angel food cake. Candy bars do not by themselves rot your teeth. It is your belief system that determines whether these foods are good or bad. That is why I experimented with the ice cream. If I had been taught from childhood that ice cream was the mainstay of my diet, then it would have no special significance. It would just be ordinary food and I would be looking for something else to make me "feel" happy. So, after 6 months of eating this diet, ice cream became just ordinary food.

What did you eat after the ice cream diet?

Nothing. I fasted for two years.

What foods make you happy?

This is precisely what I learned on the ice cream diet: Happiness is not a function of food. Happiness is an inner nourishment. You bring your happiness to the dinner table. The dinner does not make you happy. However, your relationship to the dinner can support or disrupt your emotional state. If you are at peace when you begin eating and your meal causes indigestion, then you have disturbed that peace—your happiness. Food does not create happiness, but it can disturb it or support it. That is why we must carefully select what we put inside our bodies and also be careful about the manner of delivery. Eating too quickly makes poison out of the healthiest, most nutritious food. Eating when you are not hungry is like forcing yourself to drive a car when you are tired. If you are miserable while you are eating, you are not prolonging your life, you are prolonging your misery. Choose a diet that both supports your body and your happiness.

Design your eating environment. Decide: Do I want to dine alone? With friends? In a restaurant? In silence? Indoors? Outdoors? What gives you pleasure? To enjoy the process of eating is as important as selecting the food. If you are enjoying your meal, you are assimilating the vitamins and boosting your immune system. Scientists would have us believe that the immune system is supported purely by nutrients. But it is not. It is actually nourished by positive energy. When I was on my two year fast, I had no outside source of nutrients. Yet, my immune system was as strong as ever. Of course, food will contribute its nutrients, but it is your enjoyment of the food and the positive feelings around it that send the strongest message to the immune center and your overall health.

What do you eat now?

At my age, I take enormous pleasure in just breathing. But how does it serve you to know what an old man eats? The body changes with the different ages. What an infant eats is different from what a teenager eats. And an adult does not eat like a teenager. We must be in tune with the process of change. I ate only raw foods for 40 years. It served me well, but that phase is over now. My body has benefitted from and achieved what it needed from that diet. For example, I see you are now wearing a coat here on top of the mountain, but when you descend into the warmth of the valley, you will shed the coat. You must change because your circumstances change. You must leave your coat though it served you well and you are grateful for having had it.

Asking me what I eat may be a curiosity, but it will not help you discover what is best for you to eat. However, to satisfy that curiosity, I will tell you how I make my food choices. First of all, I can tell you that most of my nourishment does not come from food; it comes from love. I eat whatever people serve me when it is served with love. I have visited your fast food American restaurants where the kitchen is an assembly line, and the meals are delivered by truck, microwaved, fried, and served. There is no comparison between this food and that prepared by conscious chefs who take pride in their art and enjoyment in the feeding of others. There is a difference between vegetables grown with chemicals and those grown by farmers who nourish the soil by natural means and garden according to the rhythms of the land. There is a difference when a chef chooses the fresh vegetable over the wilted one. Even if the chef puts in too much sugar, it cannot hurt when that treat is prepared with joy.

How do we know if our diet is fulfilling our nutritional needs?

This is a big problem. Not the getting of our nutritional needs—that is easy. The problem is that our knowledge is getting in the way. Modern science has provided us with wonderful information about food. Thanks to science, we know all about vitamins and proteins, and the tiny molecules that are contained within. But did you know that 100 years ago, no one knew about vitamins? So, how did they figure out what to eat? Imagine, for thousands of years, people ate without knowing anything about vitamins! Today, we have charts and books describing the vitamins in every bite we take. All the food on the shelves in your American supermarkets has its nutrients listed and quantified. People even go to nutritionists to learn how to nourish themselves. They buy an armful of supplements and attempt to juggle the various nutrients into the correct combinations to attain perfect health. But I tell you, even with our modern scientific apparatus, we do not have the capacity to orchestrate the thousands of chemicals in food into the correct arrangement for health. Maybe you throw in a little vitamin A, some vitamin C, a little B1, B2, B12, E, K, F....But, do you really know what you are doing? It is a gambling game.

....Even with our modern scientific apparatus, we do not have the capacity to orchestrate the thousands of chemicals in food into the correct arrangement for health.

A symphony may be composed of a million notes, but it has only twelve tones. These twelve tones are played in different combinations and speeds, with repetitions and punctuation which, in the hands of an artist, becomes beautiful music. But imagine having those 12 notes in your cupboard. You know how beautiful they can be, so you take lots of them and attempt to put them in order. But a symphony is not a scientific order. Knowledge of the specific tones and their effects will not enable you to replicate the beautiful music that resonates in a healthy body. It cannot be done with the conscious mind.

So it is with food. Man cannot duplicate the wisdom of nature and that includes the natural forces inside our bodies. You cannot orchestrate the thousands of different chemicals and their relative amounts in your body. That job should be left to your innate intelligence. The little seed knows how to grow into a big plant. You may attempt to point its roots to the ground or tug on its leaves to help it grow, but it would be best to just feed it water.

When it comes to your health, the best thing to do is to become a good listener. The more closely you listen, the better you will flow with the music of perfect health. Tune into your body, not with a microscope, but with closed eyes. Listen to your stomach, feel your heart, and connect with each meal before your eat it.

People are striving to achieve better health through diet. But if health is a rainbow, then diet is only one of the colors. For many people, health means: "I am not in pain." But health is more than the absence of disease. It is an attitude: He was at ease; he "dis-turbed" that ease; now, he is "dis-eased." If you are seeking to achieve health through diet, you must develop a healthy relationship with food and a healthy attitude in your life. There is no perfect diet. When you sit down to eat, half the meal is about the food and the other half is about the feelings you bring to it. If you are fearful while you are eating, then you are eating fear. If you are miserable, you are prolonging your misery. This is true even if your plate is filled with the finest organic foods.

If you are looking to get healthy from food, you must develop a healthy relationship with food and a healthy attitude in your life. There is no perfect diet.

So, attitude is another color of the rainbow. You can eat the best diet and still be miserable. In fact, some people fuss over their diet so much, it adds to their misery. You may die early in life because of your misery and in spite of your good diet. On the other hand, you have probably heard of people who smoke, and drink liquor, and live well into their nineties. Doctors have proven that smoking and drinking kills and many middle-aged people have died from these addictions. But these others are alive and well at ninety! Why? So now we must consider other factors. I would ask: What is your attitude when you smoke? Do you smoke as a reaction to stress or just for enjoyment? Attitude is your salvation. That is why the "placebo" pill cures so many people. It is just sugar, but the patient believes it can cure him, so it does. So, what you think and feel has a greater effect on what you eat than the food itself.

You mentioned vegetarianism. Is it the best diet?

We do not wish to kill any conscious beings. That is violence and violence makes the world a harsh place. Go to a zoo. Look at the animals. The carnivores are prowling and growling. They are restless and angry. Now look at the sheep, the cows, the horses and elephants. They sit in peace and eat from your hand.

As soon as you kill something it decays. Decaying matter creates poisons in your body. You have to work hard to counteract these poisons. Flesh also takes more time to digest. By the time you have digested meat and counteracted its poisons, you have spent more energy than you have gained from eating it. But a vegetable is easy to digest. When you eat vegetables and fruits, you are eating matter that is still alive. The vegetable cells contain living nutrients that your body can utilize in its own tissues and cells.

You can eat half a potato, put the other half back in the ground and you will get more potatoes. Try this with a piece of meat and see what you get.

But aren't you also killing the vegetables?

Yes, but it is not the same as killing animals. The vegetable kingdom is here to serve us. When you pick a fruit, the tree remains unharmed and is ready to give more. When you harvest beans, some seed falls back to the ground and within 90 days, you have more beans. You can eat half a potato, put the other half back in the ground and you will get more potatoes. Try this with a piece of beef and see what you get.

Many people are overweight. What is your advice for overeaters?

Almost everyone eats more food than they need. Fast, and you will be amazed at your ability to function without food. A big part of eating is ritual and routine. If your ritual is three times each day, then you become accustomed to that. Here, on top of the mountain, the monks take only one meal per day. Their level of physical activity is low and the more quiet the body, the more clear the mind. We have no track runners or weightlifters here. Everybody has to regulate their consumption of food according to their physical requirements. But in Western civilization, people eat for the wrong reasons. If you eat out of boredom or depression, that food serves no bodily function. So it piles up. It is a simple law: burn it, or store it. Why do you think so many people have bad breath? Food, eaten in excess of the body's capacity, remains in the stomach undigested. Excess eating converts our stomachs into latrines. No wonder it fouls the breath. We are carrying around a cesspool inside us! We have become a society of gluttons driven by our tongues, seeking evanescent sensations to fill the void created by our unhappiness. This misdirected search for happiness through food creates insanity. Some even take purgatives in order to vomit what they have eaten so that they may be able to devour more. Yes, food naturally gives pleasure. But that pleasure comes from the satisfaction of true hunger.

We have become a society of gluttons driven by our tongues, seeking evanescent sensations to fill the void created by our unhappiness.

Because of your bad habits and artificial ways of living, few people in the Western world eat for the purpose of nourishment. That is why so many are overweight. They view food as entertainment or use it to fill gaps of psychological need. Ninety percent of the people who lose weight on a diet, gain it back again within six months. Although they succeed on the physical level, the weight problem returns because they make no other changes. If you question the successful dieters, you will learn that the only possible way to lose weight, is to gain life. The successful dieter launches his program with the goal: "I want to feel better about myself. I want to be happier."

Happiness should be your goal. If not, then ask: why you are seeking health? Is it only to take pride in bodily appearance? If this is the only goal, then we will be caught in a struggle with Satan over control of our body. If we lose, then our body becomes nothing more than a filthy vessel with poisons and odors and anger oozing from every orifice and pore. Instead, strive to make your physical body an abode of God. Our body is a gift that was given to us at birth in purity and perfection. It is our duty to keep it pure, both from within and without, so that when the time comes, we can return it in the same state of beauty in which we received it. Although, we never return exactly what we take, but we do convert food, air, and water into positive energy. It is that energy that we return to all those who come in contact with us and it becomes our legacy to the world.

GLOSSARY

Absorption

The process of food being broken down into a state where it can be transported by the bloodstream.

Assimilation

The process wherein cells utilize the results of digestion. Nutrients in the bloodstream are taken in by the body's cells.

Celiac Disease

An inflammatory bowel condition in which the villi have collapsed or flattened.

Colitis

A chronic inflammation or possibly even ulceration of a section of the large intestine.

Crohn's Disease

A chronically inflamed section of the intestinal tract, usually where the small and large intestine connect.

Fermented Foods

Sauerkraut, yoghurt, seed cheese, etc., any food that is aged in the proper way to develop friendly bacteria.

FOS

Fructo-Oligosaccharides. A group of (non-digestible) Oligosaccharides composed of short-chain polymers of Fructose.

G.E.R.D.

Chronic heartburn, also known as "Gastro-Esophageal Reflux Disease."

Irritable Bowel Syndrome

Abnormal muscular contractions in the colon. A form of colitis, but without the inflammation. Symptoms, which continue for years, include intestinal cramps with constipation and/or diarrhea.

Leaky Gut Syndrome

A chronically inflamed section of villi in the small intestine that have become porous, enabling incompletely digested food particles to enter the bloodstream.

Peristalsis

The normal, healthy undulations of the intestines that move food through on its journey to the rectum.

Phytochemicals

Plant compounds that have therapeutic benefits but are not part of the more conventional proteins, minerals or alphabetic vitamins (Vitamin A, B, C, etc.). Antioxidents, bioflavinoids and cerotins are phytochemicals.

Probiotics

Friendly bacteria such as acidophilus and bifidus. While antibiotics kill off all bacteria and in the process compromise the immune system, probiotics fight bad bacteria by competing against them. There are hundreds of different strains. They are a crucial part of any digestion repair program. Available in health food stores and from your natural health practitioner.

Villi

Projections from the small intestine through which we absorb nutrients from our food.

RESOURCES

American Association of Naturopathic Physicians.
866-538-2267. Fax 202.237.8152. 4435 Wisconsin Avenue, NW,
Suite 403, Washington, DC 20016. www.naturopathic.org. Find a
naturopathic doctor (ND) in your area. They evaluate stool tests,
work with herbs, supplements, and focus on systemic causes instead of symptoms.

Genova Diagnostics. 800-522-4762. 63 Zillicoa Street,
Asheville, NC 28801. www.GDX.net. Famous for their *Compre-
hensive Digestive Stool Analysis* yielding important information
about the ecology of the GI tract, including intestinal wall integ-
rity, small bowel bacterial overgrowth, yeast presence, immune
function, parasite activity, etc. Also several other valuable tests.

Doctor's Data. 800-323-2784. www.doctorsdata.com. Lab
tests for stool, hair, blood, urine, toxic metals, amino acids, etc.

Renew Life. 866-450-1787, 813-871-3200. Clearwater, FL.
www.renewlife.com. One of the best sources of digestive health
products and information available in health food stores.

Colema Boards of California. 800-745-2446. 916-347-5868.
PO Box 1879, Cottonwood, CA 96022. www.colema-boards.com.
Manufacturer of this enema/colonic device. Founded by the
health pioneer V.E. Irons. Also sells bentonite liquid and other
colon products.

Optimal Health Network. Madison, WI. 608-242-0200.
www.enemabag.com and www.colonichealth.com. Complete
home enema supplies and colonic information.

Prime Pacific Health Innovations. North Vancouver, BC
Canada. 1-800-223-9374. 604-929-7019. www.thecolonet.com

Manufacturers of FDA registered professional and home (self-service) colonic equipment. Home Model "Colonet" comes with ultra violet sterilizer and water filter. Cost is approximately $1,000 US.

International Association of Colon Hydrotherapists. 210-366-2888. Fax 210-366-2999. San Antonio, TX. E-mail iact@healthy.net. www.i-act.org. Referral list of colon hydrotherapists in you area.

Crohn's & Colitis Foundation of America Inc. 800-932-2423 or 212-685-3440. Fax 212-779-4098. New York, NY. www.ccfa.org Support and basic education and public service programs about inflammatory bowel disease for patients, professionals, and the general public. **Pediatric Crohn's & Colitis Association Inc.** 617-489-5854. Newton, MA. www.pcca.hypermart.net.

Irritable Bowel Syndrome Association. 416-932-3311. Fax 416-932-8909. www.ibsassociation.org. Nonprofit organization dedicated to helping everyone who suffers from IBS through patient support groups, treatment, accurate information, and education.

Irritable Bowel Syndrome Self Help Group. 1440 Whalley Ave. #145, New Haven, CT 06515. www.ibsgroup.org. E-mail: ibs@ibsgroup.org. Bulletin board, library, and web links.

Gluten Intolerance Group of North America. 206-246-6652. Fax 206-246-6531. 15110 10th Avenue SW., Suite A Seattle, WA 98166-1820. www.gluten.net Provides education and support to public and professionals about celiac disease.

Celiac Sprue Association. 877-CSA-4CSA. Fax 402-558-1347. PO Box 31700 Omaha, NE 68131-0700. www.csaceliacs.org. "Celiacs Helping Celiacs" dedicated to helping individuals with celiac disease and dermatitis herpetiformis worldwide through education, research and support.

BIBLIOGRAPHY

The New Vegetarian. by Gary Null. Delta, 1978 New York.

U.S. Department of Agriculture. Agricultural Research Service. 2001. USDA Nutrient Database for Standard Reference, Release 14. Nutrient Data Laboratory.

Food Combining Made Easy. by Herbert M. Shelton. School of Natural Hygiene, 1951 San Antonio, TX.

The Oil Story. by Eva Graf. Center of the Light, 1981. Great Barrington, MA 01230.

Encyclopedia of Medicinal Herbs. by Joseph Dadans, N.D., PhD. Arco Publishing Co. 1975, New York, N.Y.

Back To Eden. by Jethro Kloss. Woodbridge Press, 1939. Santa Barbara, CA.

Dictionary Of Man's Foods. by William L. Esser. Natural Hygiene Press, 1972. Chicago, IL.

Toxicants Occurring Naturally in Foods. Strong, Frank M. National Academy of Science, 1973, pp.487-489. Chrmn, Subcommittee on Naturally Occurring Toxicants in Foods.

Food for Health. Ensminger, A.H., Ensminger, M.E., Konlande, J.E., Robson, J.R.K. Pegus Press, 1986. Clovis, California.

The Health Guide. by Mahatma Gandhi. The Crossing Press, Trumansburg, NY. 1965.

Nourishing Wisdom. by Marc David. Published by Bell Tower, Stockbridge, Mass.

The Positive Times Newsletter. by Posner, Jerry, Wescott, Don & Jacquelyn. PO Box 244, W. Stockbridge, MA 01266-0244. Subscription $10.00 per year.

Beyond Words. by Swami Satchidananda. Holt, Reinhart and Winston, New York. 1977.

Nutrition. by Rudolf Hauschka. Rudolf Steiner Press. 1967. Great Barrington, Mass.

Index

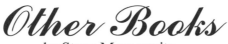

Other Books
by Steve Meyerowitz
www.Sproutman.com

Water the Ultimate Cure
Discover Why Water is the Most Important Ingredient in your Diet and Find Out Which Water is Right for You. 2001.

Power Juices Super Drinks
Quick, Delicious Recipes to Reverse and Prevent Disease. 2000.

Juice Fasting & Detoxification
Use the Healing Power of Fresh Juice to Feel Young and Look Great. 2002.

Wheatgrass Nature's Finest Medicine
The Complete Guide to Using Grass Foods & Juices to Revitalize Your Health. 2006.

Sproutman's Kitchen Garden Cookbook
Sprout Breads, Cookies, Soups, Salads & 250 other Low Fat, Dairy Free Vegetarian Recipes. 1999.

Sprouts the Miracle Food
The Complete Guide to Sprouting. 2007.

Sproutman's "Turn the Dial" Sprout Chart
A Field Guide to Growing and Eating Sprouts. 2007.

Clinician's Complete Reference to Complementary/Alternative Medicine.
Editor Donald W. Novey, MD, Steve Meyerowitz, co-author. 2000.

Food Combining and Digestion
101 Ways to Increase Stomach Power and Maximize Digestion 2008.

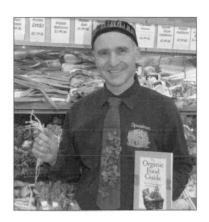

Steve Meyerowitz began his journey to better health in 1975 to correct a chronic, lifelong condition of severe allergies and asthma. After two months of eating a raw foods, vegetarian diet, his symptoms cleared. Steve endured 20 years of disappointment with conventional medicine before he restored his health through his own program of dietary purification, lifestyle adjustment, exercise, fasting, juicing and living foods.

Over the years, he has lived on and experimented with many so called 'extreme' diet/lifestyles including raw foods, fruitarianism, sprouts, dairy and flourless vegetarianism, and fasting. In 1977, he was pronounced "Sproutman" by *Vegetarian Times Magazine* in a feature article that explored his innovative kitchen gardening ideas and recipes.

After 10 years as a music and comedy entertainer, Steve made a complete lifestyle change for his health. In 1980, he opened *The Sprout House*, a "no-cooking school" in New York City. There, he began a formal program of teaching kitchen gardening and the preparation of gourmet sprouted and living vegetarian foods. Steve has invented two home sprouters, the *Hemp Sprout Bag* and the *Kitchen Garden Salad Grower*.

Steve has been featured on the *Home Shopping Network, QVC, TV Food Network,* in *Prevention, Organic Gardening* and *Flower & Garden Magazines.* Steve and his family, including three little sprouts, now live and breathe the fresh air of the Berkshire mountains of Massachusetts.